THE WOMAN WHO FOOLED THE WORLD

BELLE GIBSON'S CANCER CON, AND THE DARKNESS AT THE HEART OF THE WELLNESS INDUSTRY

Beau Donelly & Nick Toscano

SCRIBE

Melbourne • London

Scribe Publications Pty Ltd
2 John St, Clerkenwell, London, WC1N 2ES, United Kingdom
18–20 Edward St, Brunswick, Victoria 3056, Australia

First published by Scribe 2017
This edition published 2018

Typeset in 12/17pt Adobe Garamond Pro by the publishers

Printed and bound in the UK by CPI Group (UK) Ltd, Croydon
CR0 4YY

Scribe Publications is committed to the sustainable use of natural
resources and the use of paper products made responsibly from those
resources.

9781911344575 (UK paperback)
9781925322460 (Australian paperback)
9781947534063 (US paperback)
9781925548594 (e-book)

A CiP entry for this title is available from the British Library and the
National Library of Australia.

scribepublications.co.uk
scribepublications.com.au

THE WOMAN WHO FOOLED THE WORLD

Beau Donelly is a multi-award-winning journalist who covered social affairs for *The Age* and *The Sydney Morning Herald*. His news-breaking, writing, and investigative skills have been recognised by the United Nations and the Melbourne Press Club. Donelly has been awarded for an exposé on illegal brothels, coverage of clergy sex-abuse trials, and reporting on disability issues. He has also been a finalist for Australian journalism's highest honour, the Walkley Award. Donelly has a Bachelor of Journalism from Monash University, and is based in Europe.

Nick Toscano is a multi-award-winning journalist based in Melbourne, who specialises in federal politics, business workplace relations, and the labour movement for *The Age* and *The Sydney Morning Herald*. He has been awarded the Grant Hattam Quill for Investigative Journalism, and has twice received the highest honour in Australian journalism, the Walkley Award, for exposing the country's biggest-ever underpayment scandal. Toscano has a Bachelor of Arts from the University of Melbourne and a Masters in Journalism from RMIT.

For Avril

'Of all the ghouls who feed on the bodies of the dead and the dying, the cancer quacks are [the] most vicious and most heartless.'

Morris Fishbein, former editor of the *Journal of the American Medical Association*

'I gave up on conventional treatment when it was making my cancer more aggressive and started treating myself naturally. I have countless times helped others do the same, along with leading them down natural therapy for everything from fertility, depression, bone damage and other types of cancer.'

Belle Gibson

CONTENTS

THE QUEEN IS DEAD

Belle Gibson sat on a blue-cushioned pew, her sleek blonde hair pulled back and tied high in a bun. She was flanked by two women. The older woman had her arm around Gibson's shoulder; the younger one clutched her hand. Gibson, sobbing loudly, appeared as though she might collapse, were it not for their support.

It was Friday, 6 March 2015. The memorial service in Buderim, ninety minutes' drive north of Brisbane, was at Lifepointe Baptist Church, a pentagon-shaped building behind the motorway that links the city to the beaches in the north. It looked more like a mid-sized concert hall than a place of worship. There were slick light and sound systems, a stage, a mezzanine floor, and enough space for almost 1,000 people. On this autumn morning, a sea of mourners wearing colourful clothing gathered in their grief. Among the large but tight-knit circle were public-relations specialists and self-help authors, life coaches, and wellness-industry entrepreneurs.

They were here to farewell Jess Ainscough, known to her fans as 'The Wellness Warrior'. She had died at home on the Sunshine Coast the week before, aged 29, almost seven years after being diagnosed with an incredibly rare, slow-growing, and incurable cancer called an epithelioid sarcoma. In her quest to survive, Ainscough had overhauled her lifestyle, and became a devotee of the controversial Gerson Therapy (a regimen of five-daily coffee enemas, raw juices on the hour, every hour, and an organic vegetarian diet).

Ainscough was blonde, slim, clear-skinned, and photogenic, and had shot to fame by writing a blog about curing herself from cancer. A top-ranking health and wellness website, book deal, and celebrity appearances soon followed. She was, without question, Australia's best-known cancer-fighting wellness guru.

At the service, Ainscough's bereft father, Col, bade farewell to his blue-eyed daughter — he called her 'Jet' — and recounted anecdotes of her style and sincerity. Her first steps and first day of school, captured on film, flashed up on a projector screen. Guests spoke of the unending love between Ainscough and her partner, Tallon Pamenter. The pair were to have been married in just a few months' time. And, finally, former *Australian Idol* winner Wes Carr performed. Those who were there say it was a moving tribute; one filled with happy memories, moments of laughter, and smiles through the tears.

Through it all, Gibson wept, at times uncontrollably, and over the top of everyone else. 'Some guests seemed put off by it,' one remarked. 'She was noticeably having outbursts.'

'It was like she was making a point of being seen and heard,' said another. 'Like she was trying to prove that she was more devastated than everybody else who was there.'

Belle Gibson had first met Jess Ainscough in April two years before. Ainscough was addressing a Self-Love and Sisterhood conference in Prahran, a fashionable suburb in Melbourne's inner south-east. Gibson, a rising star in the self-help movement, lined up at the town hall with the scores of other fans to meet the keynote speaker after the event. Like Ainscough, she was also building an online following off the back of her story of beating terminal cancer, and was on the cusp of launching a fast-growing business.

Gibson used the opportunity to tell Ainscough about the health and wellness smartphone app she was building. The app was called The Whole Pantry. Developed over several months, it included healthy meal planners and recipes based on natural ingredients, and would go on to be downloaded an impressive 300,000 times. It wasn't long before the pair were moving in similar circles, albeit in different cities, and they regularly exchanged niceties on social media, usually in the form of gushing praise on Instagram of each other's 'wellness journey'.

But Gibson and Ainscough were not friends. That first meeting had never sat well with Ainscough, who felt uneasy — 'something was off about her,' she would later say.

Ainscough's manager, Yvette Luciano, remembers Gibson lining up to meet Ainscough again, this time in 2014, during her Melbourne book tour. She said Gibson stood out in the crowd of fans. 'There definitely was a feeling like she ... [was] trying to force something with Jess.'

And after Ainscough's death, Yvette took to social media to set the record straight: 'Beyond an Instagram comment or two,' she wrote, there was no relationship whatsoever, personally or professionally, between Ainscough and Gibson.

Gibson's decision to travel from her home in Melbourne's affluent bayside area to Ainscough's memorial on the tropical Sunshine Coast, almost 1,800 kilometres away, was something of a surprise to many at the service. Some of Ainscough's friends remember the bizarre moment when Gibson approached them as they were gathered outside under evergreen shade trees in a sea of bitumen car-parking, and insinuated herself into their grief. She was politely embraced, and comforted. Those closest to Ainscough then made the short drive back to the house that she and fiancé Tallon had shared with her father in Alexandra Headland. The two-storey property, 800 metres from the surf, was set back on a suburban street behind native rainforest. Gibson had never been there before, but she acted like she had.

Inside, she cried. She cried about Ainscough, and about her own cancer. 'She was hysterically sobbing, saying how devastated she was to lose Jess,' one of Ainscough's friends said. 'No one really knew what to do with her.' Yvette said she was confused to see Gibson. 'I didn't even know how she knew where Jess lived or how she got there.'

At one point, Gibson summoned the dead woman's fiancé into a bedroom and wept on his shoulder. She told him her heart was breaking, that she was petrified of dying the way his partner had. 'I don't know how they ended up in [the] room together,' one onlooker commented, 'but I do remember her coming out crying. If she didn't even know the girl, then what the fuck compelled her to be doing any of it?'

Tallon, Ainscough's partner, remembers that Gibson was upset and asked him for a private moment to talk. He knew who Belle Gibson was, through her social-media profile, but the service was the first time he had ever met her. She spoke about her own cancer, he recalls. 'At the time, there was so much going on that, I guess, I was just feeling sorry for her, thinking, maybe she's kind of thinking the same could happen to her.'

Anyone who was familiar with Belle Gibson would also have known about the life of Jess Ainscough. Both women led highly public campaigns of shunning conventional medicine, and of beating cancer from the brink of death through healthy living. And if you looked beyond their stylised Instagram posts, the subtleties of their stories were unmistakably similar.

Ainscough's quest to survive cancer began in 2008, when she was 22 and working in Sydney as an online editor for teen magazine *Dolly*. Lumps appeared on her left arm, and were later confirmed to be cancer. The best chance of prolonging her life, she was advised, was to amputate her arm at the shoulder. She signed the paperwork to have the operation, but, just days before surgery was scheduled, she was given another option: an isolated limb perfusion, where a high dose of chemotherapy is flooded only to the affected part of the body. Ainscough went for it, and the procedure temporarily staved off the disease. When it recurred the following year, she was again told that the only way to buy more time was to cut off her arm. Ainscough decided on a different approach. She turned down conventional medicine, and went looking for an alternative.

'The way I saw it I had two choices,' she wrote, three years before her death. 'I could let them chase the disease around my body until there was nothing left of me to cut, zap or poison; or I could take responsibility for my illness and bring my body to optimum health so that it can heal itself.'

Ainscough used Gerson therapy, named for physician Max Gerson, who had started a small practice in New York in 1938 and developed this regimen, based on the principle of detoxing the body and rebuilding the immune system with a clean diet, and vitamin and mineral supplements. But since the Second World War, the treatment has been dismissed as useless by health authorities around the world. Australia's National Cancer Institute's advice is that it 'cannot be recommended'. Ainscough believed otherwise. She believed it had the power to cure cancer.

She started blogging about her experience in 2010, around the time she travelled to a Gerson clinic in Mexico. Thousands of followers, mostly young women, flocked to *The Wellness Warrior,* which would become one of Australia's most popular health and wellness websites. (At one point, Ainscough claimed to have more than 2.5 million online visitors.) Ainscough believed in a conspiracy between drug companies and governments that put profit over finding a cancer cure. She said Gerson Therapy and other treatments, such as New Age mind-body interventions, offered cancer patients a *real* cure. She wrote about shunning conventional medicine, about her 'cancer recovery story', about how she was 'healing my body naturally'. She announced on her blog that she had cured herself of cancer. 'I saved my own life,' she said. Her followers pledged their solidarity, and some declared that they were following her path to treat their own cancers. 'You are such an inspiration!' one posted. 'I was recently diagnosed and am on week six of the Gerson Therapy. I also spent time at the clinic in Tijuana. I am excited [to be] on this journey to wellness and start my day by reading your words.'

Said another: 'You're living proof that cancer can be cured using natural means and good disposition.'

Ainscough went on to launch an online lifestyle guide. The two-minute promotional video features Ainscough meditating at sunset and walking along the beach with a backing track of gentle acoustic guitars. She hosted a web TV series on wellness, called 'healthtalks', in which she demonstrated, among other things, how to perform a coffee enema. She graduated from the holistic health coaching course at New York's Institute for Integrative Nutrition, and then hit the motivational speaking circuit. By 2013, Ainscough had gained national fame as the author of *Make Peace With Your Plate*, a 256-page recipe book detailing her 'healing journey' and metamorphosis from 'self-confessed party-girl and cancer patient to wellness warrior'.

The book flew off the shelves — sales topped 10,000 copies quickly. When it was released, publicity for the book declared that Ainscough was 'cancer-free'. Publisher Hay House still describes Ainscough as 'thriving'. She was neither. But it was a good story.

All the while, Ainscough was clashing with the medical community. She was being lambasted as being part of a dangerous new wave of health gurus promoting alternative therapies that claim to do more than they can. Doctors and cancer specialists were among those to speak out — not against her right to choose her own treatment, but over fears she might influence others who were desperately ill to shun potentially life-saving medicine in favour of unproven alternatives.

Ainscough's biggest supporter, her mother, Sharyn, was diagnosed with breast cancer after her daughter. She, too, rejected conventional treatment and leapt head-first into Gerson Therapy, as her daughter had done. But it didn't work, and Sharyn died. By the 2014 New Year, just as Ainscough's five-city Australian book tour was getting underway, her condition deteriorated. Later that year, she told her fans the cancer had become more aggressive after her mother's death. In her final blog post, Ainscough wrote about turning back to conventional medicine: 'My beliefs have been completely shaken up and I've had to drop any remnants of fear and ego that were preventing me from exploring these options sooner,' she said. Her family has since revealed she underwent radiation treatment in a last-ditch effort to save her life.

Then there was Belle Gibson. Her story of cancer survival started in 2009. She said she was 20 years old and working in a corporate job when she started experiencing memory loss, problems with her vision, and walking difficulties. Gibson claimed her concerns were brushed aside by her doctor and that she was prescribed antidepressants. Then, not long after, she said, she suffered a stroke

2014

at work, and tests revealed she had terminal brain cancer. She said she was given four months to live.

Gibson said she endured chemotherapy and radiotherapy for two months, but decided to stop the gruelling treatment after passing out in a city park near the hospital. She started exploring the world of alternative medicine and the detoxification properties of lemons, which got her thinking about the importance of a healthy diet. Gibson then travelled the country searching for a cure, and embarked on a quest to heal herself with nutrition and holistic medicine, including 'salt, vitamin and Ayurvedic treatments, craniosacral therapy, oxygen therapy, colonics, and a whole lot of other treatments'.

And four years later, she said, what she was doing was working. She appeared on Instagram just as the photo-sharing app was becoming popular, posting as a cancer patient healing herself naturally. She tapped into something big. Her social-media profile exploded, and she quickly amassed tens of thousands of followers. From there, Gibson decided to create 'the world's first health and wellness lifestyle app'. The app was downloaded more than 200,000 times in the month of its release, and tech giant Apple came knocking at her door. Awards and international book deals followed fast. Money rolled in, and the media lapped up the story. Emerging from obscurity, Gibson had gained traction in Australia, America, and the UK in just 18 months, becoming one of the most famous wellness personalities in the world.

For years before Ainscough's death, Gibson was positioning herself as the next poster girl for holistic health and wellness. And the template she used in her story followed a similar path. On the first page of her book, Ainscough speaks about a spiral into bad habits that began when she was a teenager eating junk food and hating her 'chunky' body. The first page of Gibson's book describes a dysfunctional home life and a binge-eating, overweight teenager. Both women talked about listening to their doctors and trying conventional medicine to treat terminal cancer, but ultimately coming to the realisation of needing to trust 'my intuition'. They both said they believed it was their only option. Ainscough said her journey of 'research and empowerment ... ultimately saved my life'. Gibson said she 'was empowering myself to save my own life'. The 'whole' way of eating, 'whole body' wellness, and 'whole life' are littered throughout the pages of their books and transcripts of interviews. Ainscough called herself a cancer survivor, and said she was 'living proof of the body's ability to heal itself', while Gibson knew her cancer was 'curable; my immune system is just suppressed'.

There was one problem, however, with Gibson's story: she didn't have cancer at all. Ainscough's illness was real, and her recipe for commercial success was indisputable, and tried and tested. She had proved it was possible to forge a wellness career from a terminal-cancer diagnosis. But in the end it was short-lived. The queen of wellness was dead now. Her website would soon be taken down. There was a void left in the market, and plenty of people ready to believe again.

Perhaps, as Belle Gibson sat in the bedroom with Tallon that day, her tears were all for show. Perhaps they were genuine, or perhaps they were about something else entirely. One thing was for certain, though: Gibson was coming undone. She knew she was about to be exposed. It was the day before Ainscough's service that we called her from *The Age* newsroom in Melbourne to discuss the myriad discrepancies in the stories of cancer and philanthropy that she had used to promote her global brand. We had been looking into her for weeks, suspicious about the veracity of her tale. Her cancer story seemed farfetched, and her claims of donating huge amounts of money to charities didn't hold water. Her phone was off. We called her partner, Clive Rothwell, who said she was on a flight to the Sunshine Coast for the service. So we typed out a list of 21 questions, asking for evidence of her cancer diagnosis and charitable donations, and seeking clarification of other parts of her story that didn't stack up, such as her age, and her qualifications.

We mentioned our deadline — 2.00 pm the following day — and then hit 'Send'.

Not long after, Gibson called back and left a message. She sounded very young. Her tone was friendly, professional, busy: 'Good afternoon. My name's Belle Gibson. I've had a missed call from you, so, if you could give me a call back that'd be great. Thank you.' Later, Gibson emailed to say she was attending the funeral of 'a close friend and someone who mentored me through many years'. She has never taken or returned our calls since. By the same time the following week, the cracks in Gibson's story would become chasms.

2

THE WOMAN WHO FOOLED THE WORLD

The extraordinary story of the woman who fooled the world begins in the decidedly ordinary suburbs of Brisbane's eastern beaches. The beaches aren't known for swimming, though; mangroves cover the shoreline, and mudflats emerge when the tide dips low. The mouth of the Brisbane River cuts into the land from Moreton Bay, separating the once working-class suburb of Wynnum from the city's international airport. On the Wynnum side of the river are a busy container port, Caltex's 50-year-old oil refinery, and a Wastewater Treatment Plant. The smell of decaying mangroves, like rotten eggs, rises up late in the afternoons. This is the suburb of wide streets and weatherboard homes, about 20 kilometres east of the city, where Annabelle Natalie Gibson grew up.

She lived here with her older brother, Nick, and her mother, Natalie, in a single-storey, gabled brick veneer on Louis Street. The house is owned by the Department of Housing and Public Works, which runs Queensland's social-housing program. Today, as investors are lured closer to the waterfront, and entire streets in Wynnum get a facelift, the three-bedroom house Gibson grew up in still stands out. Three old Fords are parked out the front, one lying on the lawn with its bonnet up under a leafy tree with pink flowers. A bright-red unregistered ute sits in the driveway, next to a rusting trailer and a refrigerator.

Wynnum was a neighbourhood beset by pockets of poverty, and has been afflicted by above-average unemployment levels. It has had a problem with armed robberies, and, to some degree, it still does. A spate of liquor store hold-ups in recent years led to local police enforcing an unusual ban on 'hoodie' jumpers. Locals, especially businesses, are trying hard to change Wynnum's image and lure tourists to the area. The suburb's new moniker, *Brisbane's Seaside*, has been printed onto brightly coloured bumper stickers.

In magazine interviews at the height of her fame, Gibson shared poignant memories of hardship from her childhood here: as a six-year-old standing on a chair, reaching over the stovetop to cook meals for her older brother; being thrust into the role of the family's primary carer; and carrying the burden of responsibility for all the housework and shopping because her mother was too sick. She describes a complicated and neglected childhood, one where she was left to fend for herself and was denied toys. 'I grew up in a dysfunctional home,' Gibson writes in her book. 'I never knew my dad, and grew up with my mum, who had multiple sclerosis, and my brother, who was autistic. Because mum was so ill, she needed a lot of help.'

Gibson rarely invited friends over to her house. Some remember seeing her older brother once or twice, but not one said they had met her mother. 'There was always an excuse as to why I couldn't,' a friend said. 'She knew my family well, but I never knew hers.' Gibson, who is estranged from her mother, says she moved out of home when she was 12 years old. 'I was, at times, begging for her to be my mother rather than the opposite way around,' she told one interviewer. Gibson's family maintains that what she has said about her childhood are barefaced lies, albeit innocuous ones in the greater scheme of things. But maybe it was lies like this that convinced a young girl she could get away with anything.

Growing up, Gibson was resilient. In the space of three years, she went to three different primary schools. Teachers described her as attentive and conscientious, and said she always did her homework. Gibson's grade-six report card calls her 'cooperative, friendly and well-mannered ... a pleasure to have in class'. By the seventh grade, she was enrolled at Wynnum Central State School. It was here where the young Gibson seemed to have really thrived. School records show that, not long after arriving, she was made school captain, and went on to win a string of awards. She was said to be an all-rounder, and a particular high-achiever in literacy. The primary-school principal remarked she was an 'exemplary' pupil whose behaviour set a good example to her peers and younger schoolmates. According to her application to the local high school, in December 2003, Gibson belonged to a youth group run by the Seventh-day Adventist Church. It also said that she cooked and cleaned for elderly residents in the neighbourhood, was involved in fundraising activities for her primary school, and volunteered for the Breast Cancer Foundation.

Gibson was accepted to Wynnum State High, the co-ed public school about a 15-minute walk from her house. She has claimed to have been severely overweight as a child, although she looks perfectly healthy in school photographs from these years. As a teenager, she was tanned and slender, with hazel-green eyes and a winning smile. Early high-school pictures reveal a girl with honey-blonde hair that hung in a long ponytail over her shoulder. By year 10, her hair was cropped, her eyebrows sculpted. Later, she went through an 'emo' phase and mixed with the local skater crowd. Gibson would get dressed up with her friends and catch the train into the city. They'd go shopping, and eat fast food and hang out on Queen Street.

Gibson said she studied hospitality and management while at school. She landed a job working part-time in sales for catering supply company PFD Food Services. It had a warehouse in the nearby industrial suburb of Lytton, where semi-trailers pull off the motorway to pick up stock, then head back out along roads burnt with black tyre marks. According to her old employer, and confirmed by her family, at one point she moved in with a local man, who also worked at the food company, and his two sons. Different people who knew her at this time put his age at between 40 and 60. No one seems to know why Gibson lived there, and no one appears to have questioned the curious living arrangement at the time. One former friend said she moved out of her mum's place when she was a teenager and into a small, two-storey house in the nearby suburb of Lota. Gibson might have lived with someone else, the friend recalls, but she never met them. She and Gibson would mostly hang out downstairs by themselves, drinking and talking.

'Where there was some type of guardian thing, I don't know,' says Jenny McDonald, who runs the nearby Manly Hotel, a family-owned pub and bistro with a gaming lounge on Wynnum's main drag. She briefly employed Gibson at the restaurant, and remembers that the teenager wasn't living with her family at the time.

Gibson had a love of acting, and enrolled in classes run by the Mercury Youth Theatre, at the local St Peter's parish hall. 'She was quite good, actually,' one of her old drama teachers remembers. Another teacher, Brendan Glanville, recalls that she also attended acting camps run by his Australian Acting Academy. In her circles in Wynnum, Gibson was known as a storyteller. But she was quickly earning herself a name for spinning stories that were nothing but fairy tales. Those who knew her describe a melodramatic girl with a tendency to imitate others, who was prone to lying. She'd say things about her life and about her family that seemed totally unbelievable. Over the years, she told a number of people that she was in a witness-protection program. One classmate recalls Gibson claiming she was a test-tube baby. 'We all felt like none of her stories she told us were true,' she says. Margaret Weier, who started high school with Gibson in 2004, said that, after having lunch with Gibson a few times at school, 'it was clear that she was a pathological liar'. Another classmate said Gibson's supposed health crises were part of an attempt to keep a boyfriend at the time.

A pattern evolved from these early years. Gibson would tell her friends and workmates stories of bogus medical dramas. First, it was her heart. It is said that she often recounted in detail how she had suffered major heart problems, that she had undergone a series of life-saving operations. 'Her story has changed multiple times over the years she told it,' said Kelsey Gamble, who went to a neighbouring school but attended drama classes with Gibson, and mixed in the same social circles. 'In our hometown, she was extremely well-known for what basically amounts to compulsive lying. She was honestly a laughing stock half the time … people made fun of her.' Kelsey was friends with Gibson on Facebook until 2014, when she wrote a public Facebook message accusing her of lying, and was blocked.

Dianne Karger remembers Gibson as a bully who didn't have many female friends in high school. 'She used to hang out with the skater boys,' recalls Dianne. 'She wasn't the nicest girl. She used to make girls cry … used to call them names.'

One of Gibson's former boyfriends said she 'couldn't go five minutes without making up a story', and so he simply started ignoring her. 'Back then it was about her heart,' said Jacob. 'It all just went over the top of my head because it was that frequent.' Jacob, who dated Gibson for a few months until she moved interstate, said she once told him the government was going to pay her $10,000 a week to look after her autistic brother. 'That's how she works,' he says. 'She just opens her mouth and starts saying stories.'

On the internet, though, something different was starting to happen. In a chat room about rock band The Flaming Lips, her stories of astonishing medical miracles were beginning to be believed. There were some doubters, but also huge outpourings of sympathy and support. Here, Gibson's biggest, most prolific, and most dangerous lie was born. 'As early as 2005, she started sharing information with me and posting in general forums on the board that she was suffering from brain cancer,' said Jason Klemm, who used to chat online with Gibson. 'I couldn't help but believe she was truly suffering from something horrible.'

In 2008, in her final year, Gibson dropped out of school. She was 16. Looking at a map of Australia, there is no place further away from Wynnum than Perth. And that's where she went, crossing the country to Western Australia, more than 4,000 kilometres away. She settled in the city, and found a job with private health insurer HBF. The company has a record of her working in its call centre for seven months until 5 January 2009. Gibson worked on the phones, listening to policyholders calling up to detail their various injuries and illnesses. A former friend says she knew Gibson in 2009, while she was working in the call centre and living in Duncraig, a northern suburb of Perth. She said Gibson was dating her friend's brother at the time. 'Back then she was telling people she had a terminal brain tumour,' she said. 'I didn't believe it. Someone with terminal brain cancer isn't going to work at a call centre every day.'

Gibson's grandmother hasn't had much to do with her since she was very young, but they used to talk on the phone. Every now and then, she would post a $5 note folded inside a letter so her granddaughter could buy herself a coffee down at Fremantle with her new friends. In a telephone conversation, the grandmother recalls, Gibson once told her that she was on a waiting list for a heart operation in Sydney with Dr Charlie Teo, a well-known neurosurgeon.

By May 2009, Gibson was crude-talking and had long, black-dyed hair. She was posting comments on a skateboarders' chat forum of mostly boys, and regularly divulging a litany of catastrophic medical problems she claimed to be suffering from. The posts became more and more incredible. She wrote not only about being treated for cancer and undergoing major surgery, but described dying on the operating table and finding bruises on her chest from the paddles that were supposedly used to shock her back to life.

'I just woke up out of a coma type thing,' she said. 'The doctor comes in and tells me the draining failed and I went into cardiac arrest and died for just under three minutes.'

In another post, she said: 'I had fluid in the pericardium (sac around heart) that needed to be drained or else my heart would've stopped pumping blood, and would've died. And I need to get a valve replaced, but can't afford it yet.' Gibson wrote about preparing for chemotherapy, more tests on her heart, rehabilitation after a 'cardiac arrest'. She also claimed, in 2009, that she had a bad reaction to the Gardasil cervical cancer vaccine, which resulted in headaches, blurred vision, slurred speech, and what she believed to be a stroke. Later, during a visit back to Brisbane, she would tell friends that her brain cancer was caused by the vaccine. By then there was a little shaved patch on the side of her head. But there was no scar.

It was on internet forums and chat rooms that the fantasy world which Belle Gibson created started to take hold. She had grown up in a generation that documents their lives online — a world where information and misinformation, real news and fake news, are sometimes impossible to distinguish — and the digital footprints she left behind cannot be erased. That said, tracing the *real* life of Gibson has not been easy. There are whole periods, many months at a time, where there is no record of her at all.

What is known is that Gibson was born in Launceston, Tasmania, on 8 October 1991. Her mother, Natalie Dal Bello, is a divorcee from Melbourne who moved around the south-eastern states of Australia before settling in Adelaide, and remarrying in 2012. Gibson's father is unknown. Natalie has described him as a 'sperm donor'. According to Gibson's grandmother, he was a nice young man from Tasmania. Gibson has an older brother. She also has half-siblings, but all our attempts to talk to them have been met with silence.

Gibson did not inherit her father's name. She was born Annabelle Smillie, after her mother's side, before Natalie changed their surname by deed poll. Gibson's maternal grandfather was a book buyer for a department store. Her great grandfather, a Scottish immigrant, was a senior constable in Victoria Police who, throughout his career, was commended for his courage and zeal. When Gibson was young, Natalie uprooted the family, and moved interstate. They had stints in Queensland, living in public housing in Strathpine, north of Brisbane, and on the coast, in Maroochydore, before finally settling in Wynnum when Gibson was 11 years old.

Since leaving Wynnum, Gibson has never stayed in one place for very long. She is estranged from her family, and has scant few long-term friends. But the ones she has kept are loyal to her. The father of Gibson's child has remained silent, and her current partner, the few times he spoke to us, chose his words very carefully. When everything began to unravel, in March 2015, just two people came to Gibson's defence. One, at first, believed in her. 'She was an amazing friend to me when my younger brother passed away from cancer,' the friend wrote to us. 'She is one of the most authentic people I have ever met.' When we contacted this person later, for this book, she told us she wanted nothing to do with it: 'These comments [were] before everything came to a head.' The other person who came out in defence of Gibson was an old school friend. She had known Gibson since they were 13 years old. 'I can assure you, her credibility is strong,' she said. 'I have known her through her childbirth, cancer diagnosis, and treatment, and the birth of The Whole Pantry app. She has been dealt a rough hand and has since been able to change that potential victim energy into a positive healing message.' She did not want to talk further.

Countless more people, however, came forward to describe Belle Gibson as a liar and a manipulator. Not a single member of Gibson's family came to her defence. Most of the people who knew Belle Gibson as the cancer survivor and app developer refuse to talk about her. The one common thread among the people she grew up with, the entourage that followed her around when times were good, and the multinational companies that partnered with her, is that none of them now wants to be associated with her or The Whole Pantry in any way. In response to questions, they either said nothing at all, pleaded to be left out of the stories, or threatened legal action.

Most of the then glowing endorsements of Gibson from other young wellness entrepreneurs have vanished, now deleted from the internet. Even some of the uncritical media coverage has disappeared. Gibson herself scrubbed every one of her social-media profiles clean — purging thousands of personal and business-related posts, and even more comments — in a matter of days.

But some things cannot be so easily deleted. In her book, Gibson says she was diagnosed with terminal brain cancer in June 2009, when she was aged 20 (she was, in fact, only 17 years old in June 2009):

I had known for a while that something didn't *feel* right, but when I saw the doctor, he told me to ignore what I was experiencing and to trial antidepressants. I tried them but they made no difference, so I went off them and went back to the doctor. I told him, 'I'm having trouble reading and seeing; sometimes walking is hard and remembering has become difficult.' All he said was, 'You work too hard, you're looking at a computer all day and you're socially isolated. Let's get your eyes tested and start that medication I gave you again.' At this point I could have taken control of my own life and got a second opinion, but instead of listening to my body and trusting my intuition, I put my faith in one 'professional.' I felt like I had hit a brick wall.

Soon afterwards I had a stroke at work — I will never forget sitting alone in the doctor's office three weeks later, waiting for my test results. He called me in and said 'You have malignant brain cancer, Belle. You're dying. You have six weeks. Four months, tops.' I remember a suffocating, choking feeling and then not much else.

Gibson later claimed that the doctor who diagnosed her in 2009 was a man named Mark Johns, whom she met at a film screening in Perth. She said he was a neurologist and immunologist from the Peter MacCallum Cancer Centre in Melbourne, who treated her initially in her share house in Perth and then later, during 2010 and 2011, in Melbourne. She said she was tested with 'electronic diagnosis equipment', a machine she described as an 'old-fashioned hard-drive with lights and metal sheets that you sat on'. She said the treatment, which she believed to be radiotherapy, was administered weekly at first, and then on a continuously intermittent basis for at least 18 months. She also claims that Mark gave her the oral chemotherapy drug Temodal. No supporting documentation proving Dr Mark Johns exists has ever been found. There is no record of him being employed by Peter Mac, or registered with the Australian Health Practitioner Regulation Agency.

Soon after Gibson said she was diagnosed, she packed up and left Perth. She claimed she moved to Melbourne to be closer to her doctor. But her grandmother believes she went to Adelaide first, and her mother says she flew back across the country, east, to Port Macquarie, on the coast of New South Wales.

As she boarded her flight out of Perth, Gibson posted a photo online looking out through the window over the wing of the aircraft and into the clouds. 'For all you pretty people missing my not so pretty face,' Gibson wrote. Wherever she was going, what is certain is that, by late 2009, Gibson was 18 years old, pregnant, and a long way from home.

3

THE BIRTH OF 'HEALING BELLE'

When Belle Gibson resurfaced online, in early 2010, it was on a parenting forum on a website called *What To Expect*. In one of her first posts, the expectant mum said she was worried because she wasn't showing yet; because she didn't 'look pregnant'. Gibson asked other mums who were due around the same time to share photos of their bumps. Later, she talked excitedly about her upcoming antenatal appointment at the Royal Women's Hospital in Parkville. She once described being brought to tears while on the phone to the baby's father, who was interstate, and she felt a kick. The baby's father is Nathan Corbett, a tradesman in his 20s who is from a beachside town in New South Wales. Gibson said she met Nathan through friends while she was living in Perth. She has always described him as her best friend. She wrote online that she had been putting off the ultrasound to determine the gender of the baby until Nathan moved to Melbourne to be with her. Then, on 9 March, when she was six months' pregnant, she finally posted the results of the scan: 'WE'RE HAVING A BOY!'

The posts on this forum have since been deleted, but the person who introduced herself as Belle, a young woman new to the city of Melbourne, had the same email address that Gibson previously used. She wrote about having cancer, detoxing, and chiropractic treatment. She said that half a Panadol tablet affected her severely and that she wouldn't get into a warm bath after 'learning about the chemicals you absorb from unfiltered water'. She wrote about her fear of miscarrying, although there were no physical signs that anything was wrong with her baby. Gibson didn't just open up about her pregnancy and her health; she also shared intimate details online about her finances, moving out of a share house, and her deep disappointment in her friends. The forum seemed to be less of a parenting resource than it was a place for a lonely young woman to connect.

On 20 April, Gibson posted about having no support network around her. She said she was cancelling her baby shower, scheduled a month before the birth, because no one had bothered to make plans to travel to Melbourne to see her. She'd tried to organise dates that suited everyone, and had even emailed them flight specials.

'They all want to come down, but have made no effort to come down for my shower date,' she wrote:

> I'm really quite upset, even depressed at seeing all of you girls organising your gorgeous showers, I'm happy for you all, and I really do hope I'm not raining down on your parades at all :) but as a first time, young mother, that has overcome a lot for this little man in me, I would love nothing more than to somewhat celebrate with my close friends and even be supported in some way by them. Because at the moment, I'm working part time, going to hospital at least once a week after work hours, then travelling an hour home to cook and clean and try and fit some rest in. I know it doesn't

sound like I'm struggling. But doing it all on your own, with all the medical dramas I've tried to fight before falling pregnant makes this so hard and was looking forward to my shower SO MUCH!

At one point, Gibson disclosed her biggest fear: not being ready to have the baby. She confessed she was scared she wouldn't be able to cope. 'I just hope that I can afford this little man,' she said, 'because right now I'm having my doubts. People are "joking" that he'll be sleeping in the dresser. I'm not usually financially strained, but it's seeming obvious that I'm underprepared.'

Gibson's son, Olivier Corbett — everyone calls him Oli — was born in July 2010. He had his mother's eyes. Nathan relocated to Melbourne, and the young family rented a unit in a motel-style block of apartments on Westbury Street in St Kilda East. According to Gibson's mother, Nathan struggled to find work and, when Oli was about one, he stayed home while Gibson got a job in a baby store. Court documents show that by the end of 2011, Gibson worked part-time, about 10 hours a week, managing a shop on Chapel Street. She still lived with Nathan then, but, by early 2012, the couple had split up. Gibson continued to refer to Nathan as her best friend, and said he still played a big part in their son's life.

After Nathan moved out, one of Gibson's friends from Brisbane came down and stayed with her and Oli in the little flat. 'I came home a few times to her in bed saying she had a cancer therapy or [an] appointment and it made her really ill.' The living arrangement didn't last long. The lease was soon up. The friend left, and Gibson and Oli moved around the corner, to the neighbouring suburb of Caulfield North, in the heart of Melbourne's orthodox Jewish community. Theirs was a simple two-bedroom unit in a 1960s-style block of flats, which Gibson rented from a doctor and his barrister wife. It was in these rooms that she worked away on her idea for a food and wellness smartphone app.

Rebecca Jones met Gibson through a natural-parenting group that she ran in Melbourne. Gibson was a member on Facebook, but they soon caught up in person. The first time they met, at a Christmas party at Richmond Learning Centre, Gibson brought homemade banana-and-chocolate pops for the group. Everyone raved about them. She described Gibson as warm and overly friendly from their very first encounter. 'It was full on,' Rebecca recalls. 'She seemed like she already knew me. Like, she said, "I love you" the first time she met me as she was leaving.'

The Facebook group became a place for Gibson to connect with other young parents in Melbourne. She'd buy wooden toys for Oli through a local co-op that Rebecca ran. And she always tried to make a good impression with the other parents, most of whom were older than her. Once, at a mutual friend's child's birthday party, Rebecca said Gibson spent the entire time acting like the host, pouring drinks for her children, even though they were both guests. Soon, the Facebook group became a place for Gibson to workshop her business plan. When it came time to pick a name for her business, she put up a post asking the parents to brainstorm ideas.

At the start of 2012, Instagram was little more than a year old and still a profitless start-up, but it was growing, and growing fast. The photo-sharing app is now owned by Facebook and, at the time of writing, it had more than 700 million users worldwide. Belle Gibson joined Instagram before 'Instafamous' was a thing; before you could be paid tens of thousands of dollars to share a photo or sign lucrative deals with major brands if you had enough followers. When Belle Gibson was a broke, single mum who installed Instagram on her smart phone, there was no reference to social media when you looked up the word 'influencer' in the dictionary.

Just like she had done on the internet forums years before, when Gibson made her debut on Instagram, she started posting about her health. Straightaway, she claimed to be healing herself of terminal brain cancer. She had been telling people for a long time that she had been, but an MRI scan a little over a year earlier was irrefutable. In October 2011, Gibson had been referred by Dr Mark O'Reilly from the Prahran Market Clinic for a neurological assessment at The Alfred hospital. She'd reported problems with her sight, eye pain, slurred speech, and memory loss. Gibson went back with Oli, then 15 months old, to get her results, and was told everything was fine. The letter from the neurology unit registrar back to her GP makes no mention of brain cancer: 'I showed Annabelle the images today and reassured her that the results were perfectly normal.'

When she created her Instagram account, Gibson chose a handle that was unambiguous: *healing belle*. Her bio read, 'Belle Gibson: Gamechanger with brain cancer + a food obsession'. From her phone she uploaded a stream of stylised photos of what she was eating and doing during the day. Her feed evolved into posts about the benefits of different 'superfoods', living naturally, and getting back to basics. She copied and pasted inspirational quotes from the internet, such as, 'Stop waiting for Friday, for summer, for someone to fall in love with you, for life. Happiness is achieved when you stop waiting for it and make the most of the moment you're in now.' And: 'Respect yourself enough to walk away from anything that no longer serves you, grows you, or makes you happy.' And: 'Your dreams belong to you. Remember that.'

There were recipes for organic meals and healthy juices. Photos of perfect-looking food. Lemon tea served in beautiful china. Spreads of paw paw, raspberries, and passionfruit. A pastel-coloured chart with pictures of foods that help hydrate. An outstretched hand holding a freshly cut coconut over cerulean-blue water in a tropical-looking location.

Sometimes she would post artful shots of her little boy playing in an old train yard, or displaying his artwork, or drinking a 'hemp super smoothie' out of a vintage jar. Other times, they were of her; a softly lit selfie in front of the bathroom mirror, or just generally radiating health and happiness. She was lithe and photogenic. Gibson gave advice about treating various medical conditions naturally. She wrote about her cancer and other health scares she experienced. But no matter how bad she made it sound, Gibson *always* looked the picture of health. She had youth and beauty and a bit of edge. In one close-up photo, taken in the car, Gibson wears oversized sunglasses and a nose ring. She has pink-pursed lips and perfect skin. 'I feel like I'm dying … and I'd know,' she captioned the post.

Gibson's online persona was always inspiring. She framed cancer in a way it hadn't been framed before. She gave her fans a glimpse of life with a terminal disease, and what she showed them was *living*. Looking in from the outside, her world was one full of happiness, hope, spirit, glamour. Gibson reinvented herself as the avatar of 'wellness'. And just like that, a new wellness warrior was born on social media. It was the perfect forum for attracting an army of adoring devotees.

Only a few months into her new venture, Gibson took to her @ TheWholePantry Facebook account to post: 'I have been healing a severe and malignant brain cancer for the past few years with natural medicine, Gerson therapy and foods,' she proclaimed. 'It's working for me and I am grateful to be here sharing this journey with over 70,000 people worldwide.'

Gibson would later tell her publisher that she believed her legions of online followers were attracted to her because what she was doing 'was so raw and authentic'. There was not enough honesty out there, she claimed, and here she was, sharing her deeply personal story. 'I think too many people on social media overly "edit" themselves,' Gibson said. 'Right from the start I was very open, and treated Instagram as my personal space — I really think it was that authenticity that people were attracted to.'

Whatever it was about Gibson, in a very short space of time @healing_belle attracted an astonishing 200,000 followers. They were, for the most part, health-conscious young women who hung off her advice. By the hundreds, they lavished her with praise in the comments sections of her Instagram photos, saying they felt deep connections with her. They called her a warrior and an angel. 'Without doubt you are THE most inspirational person I have ever encountered,' said one. 'I have never met you but I 'know' you. I have never heard you speak but I 'hear' you. I have never seen you in person but I 'look' at you in awe, in wonder and in the greatest admiration I have ever felt for anyone.'

Gibson's foray into Instagram paved the path for her commercial enterprise. In early 2013, she started recruiting her team. On 16 April, she registered the business name The Whole Pantry. A few months later, on 17 July, she registered the company Belle Gibson Pty Ltd. Its principal place of business was her little flat, Unit No. 4, on Inkerman Road in Caulfield North. But, in one of the many mistakes that would contribute to her undoing, she gave her correct date of birth when filing the paperwork. Later, Gibson opened two bank accounts for her business at ANZ's Acland Street branch in St Kilda. She didn't have her driver's licence yet, so she used her learner's permit as identification.

By now Gibson had a new partner, Clive Rothwell, an older

man originally from Adelaide, South Australia. He used to work as a consultant in the IT department for RMIT University, at Melbourne's city campus. He is a mysterious figure, whom many have speculated played an active role in the creation of The Whole Pantry and has more to answer for. But Clive has always denied having anything to do with the running of the business. While it's true that he works in IT and has experience in financial systems, Clive never had any legal control over The Whole Pantry or its bank accounts. Gibson, at all times, has been the director and sole shareholder of the company, and she was always in control of its social-media accounts.

The only paper trail between Clive and the business is the evidence that he registered and paid for the domain for Gibson's website, thewholepantryapp.com. He put down Gibson's home address, his mobile number, and his personal Yahoo email account.

Gibson said that she fell pregnant again, this time to Clive, the year before the app was launched, but lost the baby at five months. The sorrow, she writes in her book, was the impetus for starting an Instagram account:

> I needed something to break the negative cycle, and I realised there must be other people out there, feeling just as unsupported as I was, so I started posting on Instagram — I wanted to share what I had learnt about health and nutrition on my journey with cancer. I said right from the start that I was a brain cancer patient, on a quest to heal myself naturally. I was totally overwhelmed by the immediate response to my first posts — my Instagram account got ridiculous, with hundreds of people contacting me, offering advice and sharing their own stories. What I was writing about was really resonating with my community, and it still amazes me how we've all come together.

Almost immediately, Gibson got to work on building a smartphone app:

I realised that I had tapped into this whole world of unsupported, unmotivated, uninspired people and for anyone to feel like that just wasn't okay for me. I wanted to share what I had learnt on my journey with as many people as possible so I decided to create the world's first health and wellness lifestyle app. I couldn't get the vision out of my head — as soon as I had the idea I was passionately dedicated to making it happen as quickly as possible. I made sure I surrounded myself with the best team, and I funded it by drawing on old medical loans and credit cards, borrowing from friends and asking people working with me in the early days to hold off on initial invoices. I expected it to take about 18 months, but it was ready to launch after only seven months, by August 2013. If something is important enough to you, you find a way to make it happen.

Gibson has been called an app developer countless times, and, in one interview, she claimed she had learnt how to write code. What really happened, though, was that Gibson recruited a group of young developers to build The Whole Pantry app for her on the cheap. Two Swinburne University of Technology graduates, Alex Benevento and Christopher Horner, who had worked together at Collingwood app-design company Gridstone, freelanced for her on the side. According to their postings online, Chris developed the Android version while Alex built the iPhone app with a Melbourne designer named Zane David.

Zane made contact with us 48 hours after the first story about Gibson's deception was published in March 2015.

'I'll start by saying that I am not surprised she has been caught out for lying,' he wrote in an email, 'as I have always suspected her of being a pathological liar and using her cancer story to con the public.'

Zane said Gibson hired him to help *bring her idea to life*, but that he was shunned from The Whole Pantry team as soon as the app launched. He said they built the app for her at a fraction of the usual cost. 'She used her illness to ask others for a discount, to believe in her story and what she was doing, in order to help her get the message out to others,' he said. 'I now realise this was merely the start of her deception, using her illness for financial gain.'

David Glance, the director of the Centre for Software Practice at the University of Western Australia, estimates the cost of developing an app with the functionality of The Whole Pantry could very well be in the region of $50,000.

Zane said he had confronted Gibson on a couple of occasions about a string of suspected lies. He also said she was ungrateful for the hard work others had put in. That was when their relationship began to sour.

'I had emailed her about the lack of gratitude, only to be told that her cancer "made her forget things," so she forgot to say thank you. I believe she is one of the biggest manipulators I have met.'

We asked for more information about his dealings with Gibson, but Zane never responded. Alex Benevento never responded either, but that's less of a surprise. He went on to get a job with Apple. According to his LinkedIn profile, Alex was hired by the tech giant as an iOS software engineer in June 2015, three months after Gibson was exposed, and he is now based in San Jose, California. Alex had accompanied Gibson to Apple's headquarters the year before to modify the app for its Apple Watch. In little more than a year, over two dozen transactions, Gibson paid Alex almost $25,000 from her business account. A close-up photo of the pair in the US, with Alex standing behind Gibson's shoulder, shows them both with wide smiles.

The third developer, Chris, said he wanted nothing to do with the story. 'I'm just an app developer,' he said. 'Sorry, man.'

But the three developers all continue to spruik their professional involvement with the app online. Both Alex and Chris describe The Whole Pantry as their 'most notable work' on their LinkedIn profiles. Chris, who also promotes it on his website, acknowledges the controversy surrounding the app, but says, 'it stands alone as something well built and well designed'. They all use their online resumés to plug the fact that the app was named a standout on the Australian iTunes store.

The app *was* hugely popular. And if you look beyond the fact that its creator's story was untrue, the app was slick, aesthetic, easy to use. By all accounts, it was a winner.

It wasn't just app developers who Gibson enlisted to help set up and run her business for a cut-rate fee. She used her brand and faithful following to recruit and partner with young creative types and entrepreneurs from around Melbourne. She always framed it as a 'collaboration', something mutually beneficial. What it was, in fact, was discounted labour in exchange for publicity.

By the end of winter, the app was ready. On 5 August 2013, The Whole Pantry went live. It contained more than 50 gluten-free, paleo, and vegan recipes, as well as health and wellness lifestyle guides, recipe conversion tools, and a shopping-list function. The app was 'not just about food,' Gibson would later say. It was also about 'combating stress, achieving wellness and a healthy, wholesome lifestyle'. Gibson, just 21 years old, could not have anticipated the success that lay just around the corner. The Whole Pantry took off overnight, earning the No. 1 rating in the App Store in its debut month. By the end of 2013, it was named Apple's *Best Food and*

Drink App, and the second-best iPhone app in the world. It was downloaded hundreds of thousands of times globally, and inspired lucrative book deals in Australia, the US, and the UK. The Whole Pantry brand would earn Gibson half a million dollars in less than two years.

–4–

WHAT THE HELL IS WELLNESS?

Many years ago, long before Belle Gibson was credited as the creator of the world's first health, wellness, and lifestyle app, a lanky young doctor named John W. Travis went for a walk in Baltimore. He had just graduated from medical school and had moved there to complete a residency at Johns Hopkins University. Bored with much of the curriculum, he frequently visited the campus bookshop.

On this spring day, in 1972, he rummaged through the unloved paperbacks piled on a clearance table and fished out a book, *High Level Wellness*, marked down to $2.

'Wellness,' John mused, and leafed through the opening pages. He paid the shop assistant and took the book home. 'I didn't like the word at first,' he recalls, 'but I really liked the ideas. It turned out to be the best two bucks I ever spent.'

John Travis was totally gripped. *High Level Wellness* was a collection of transcribed radio talks by Halbert Dunn, the founder and chief of the US National Office of Vital Statistics from the 1930s to 1960, and an assistant surgeon-general. Dunn's concept of 'high-

level wellness' was about promoting the *positive* aspects of health —
the aspects that went beyond simply avoiding getting sick. It made
sense to the young doctor. *Wellness* was the opposite of *illness*. And
just as there were many degrees of illness, there were also many
degrees of wellness.

Just because you are not sick or showing any overt symptoms,
and you could get a check-up and obtain a clean bill of health,
explains John, 'that doesn't mean you are *well*'. You might still
be bored, depressed, anxious, or unhappy. All of this can set the
stage for physical and mental illness. Stress, for instance, is often
linked to the onset of disease. And negative emotional states can
increase smoking, drinking, and overeating. Way ahead of its time,
High Level Wellness taught that wellness was a continuing pursuit
that had a holistic approach: one of mind, body, and spirit. And
also other key factors, like the environmental, social, emotional,
intellectual.

'There was another whole dimension besides treating illness,' he
says, 'another whole dimension that medicine wasn't addressing.'

By 1975, John wanted to get out of Baltimore. He decided to
head west and return to Mill Valley, California, where he had lived
during his internship. There, he met a man named Don Ardell, the
head of the Bay Area Health Planning Agency, who, it turned out,
had also read Dunn's work and considered him a visionary.

John rented a suite of offices in a renovated building surrounded
by redwood trees on the edge of the downtown district, and opened
the world's first-ever wellness centre — the Wellness Resource Center.
He began the centre with a part-time practitioner and a shared
secretary. Meanwhile, Don Ardell was gaining national attention
touring the country speaking about wellness to hospitals and health-
planning agencies. The small centre grew to employ about a dozen
practitioners and support staff.

There was no diagnosing here, no treating, no prescribing. They didn't take insurance. It wasn't that sort of centre. What they did provide for people who came in was a battery of lifestyle questionnaires, followed by a two-hour 'wellness assessment'. Clients were then given feedback and offered a series of wellness proposals: stress reduction, nutritional counselling, fitness counselling, or a 'lifestyle evolution' group, a form of group therapy that emphasised positives. 'We counselled them,' John says, 'and we had people coming back for multiple sessions.'

While Dunn's wellness philosophy was a set of ideas without much practical application, wrote sociologist James William Miller many years later, John translated the core ideas into a concrete program. 'It involved learning relaxation strategies, self-examination, communication training, coaching to encourage creativity, improved nutrition and fitness, visualisation techniques, and the like.'

'The idea was to help clients to know themselves better, so they could take better care of themselves.'

In the following years, John Travis was featured in magazines and prime-time TV interviews. He wrote and self-published *The Wellness Workbook*, which was later picked up by a national publisher and eventually sold a quarter of a million copies. Hundreds of letters began flooding into their centre; people were hungry to find out more; nurses were asking how they could bring up such novel ideas with their doctors.

'In those early days, this wasn't something people had ever heard about ... we had to spell the word out over the phone: 'W-E-L-L-N-E-S-S',' John recalls. 'But it caught on ... and I had no idea where it was going to go.'

He didn't know it yet, but wellness was on the cusp of a tremendous transformation, soon to become a ubiquitous and big-money global economy. Before long, hospital wellness centres sprang up across the US, and then across the globe. Health practitioners started co-opting the word. Wellness treatment spas came into fashion. And so did workplace wellness programs. It even entered the lexicons of the world's largest insurance companies.

Wellness turned into a hugely popular, high-end, and fashionable pursuit, especially among society's rich and glamorous. In 2015, the wellness tourism sector was said to have generated $563 billion in revenue, and is growing by 7 per cent a year, making it the fastest-growing form of travel worldwide. According to research group SRI International, which was commissioned by the Global Spa and Wellness Summit to quantify the value of wellness tourism in 2013, more than one in six 'travel dollars' that year was spent on these kinds of holidays.

Part boot camp, part yoga retreat, the so-called 'wellness vacation' has exploded into vogue, and models and movie stars are setting the trend. Shunning the more traditional good-book-and-poolside-mojito style of getaway, the rich and famous are opting for vacations at luxury seaside wellness retreats, signing onto strict programs that are devoted to bettering body and mind. In April 2016, Australian actor Rebel Wilson was featured in *New York* magazine after posting a photo of herself on Instagram, sweating, one arm raised victoriously. She was at the end of a gruelling mountain hike in Malibu, California, where she had just done an intensive four-day 'wellness program'. The program was called Ranch 4.0, at the Four Seasons Hotel, and each day consists of a gentle wake-up with Tibetan chimes, restorative yoga, eight hours of exercise, and a 1,400-calorie organic plant-based diet.

Among other star-studded 'Ranch' alumni are A-list actors Selma Blair and Mandy Moore, who have similarly taken to Instagram with mountaintop selfies in their active wear. Not only confined to the Ranch in California, idyllic wellness retreats are flourishing across the world. Kylie Minogue and Naomi Campbell have spent holidays at the SHA Wellness Clinic, on the Spanish coast, just outside of Valencia. Russian leader Vladimir Putin was widely rumoured to have stayed here, too, on an anti-ageing and weight-loss detox diet of grains, beans, vegetables, and a daily cup of miso soup. In the Caribbean, Morgan Freeman and Emma Bunton have both reportedly travelled to BodyHoliday, a wellness-focused resort in a secluded cove on the island of St Lucia. And every year, Kate Moss goes to the LifeCo Detox and Wellness Centre in Turkey.

In 2015, according to the Global Wellness Institute, wellness trips accounted for 6.5 per cent of all tourism trips, but represented 15.6 per cent of total tourism expenditures. This, it says, is because wellness travellers come with cash to blow, spending much more money on each trip than ordinary 'non-wellness travellers'.

'Words become buzzwords,' writes Anna Kirkland in the *Journal of Health Politics, Policy and Law*, because they capture something salient about a moment in time.

In the case of 'wellness,' she says, more of us are living longer and avoiding many of the illnesses and accidents that cut short our ancestors' lives. And, in turn, the era of purely combating diseases has given way to a new ambition: *living well*. The guiding philosophy of wellness, at its core, is a deeply appealing one. In our work-obsessed lives, where smartphones and technology ensure we are forever plugged in, wellness encourages us to reflect, to reconnect with ourselves and take time to focus on our physical and mental wellbeing. Sounds good, right? But, in typical buzzword fashion, Kirkland says, wellness has come to mean 'different things to different stakeholders'. And some of those meanings are more unsettling than others.

***

These days, John Travis is exactly where you'd expect to find him: leaning back in a faded canvas deck chair, shirtless, eating cereal, in a place called Skinners Shoot, in the Byron Bay hinterland, in northern New South Wales. Home for him, for half the year, is a rusting blue-and-white caravan parked next to a banana tree in a commune with 12 other people. 'An unintentional community,' he calls it. When we met him for the first time, on a Skype video call with a two-second delay, John was kicking back on his little deck in the bush.

The combination of slow internet and piercing sun through the leaves of the poinciana tree overhead make it hard to see his face, so he shuffles around. He throws on an old purple-checkered shirt, which he leaves unbuttoned.

Even through the pixilated connection, John beams. He looks much younger than his 74 years, and radiates good health. He is grey-bearded, bald, but lean, with bright skin, clear eyes, and a toothy smile.

He chuckles, and shakes his head. 'You know, I almost gave up on the word completely.'

Wellness, John says, has devolved, stripped of much of its original meaning. It's commonplace now to hear the word used to peddle products of all descriptions, which have a tenuous link at best with personal health and wellbeing. Go into just about any pharmacy, or supermarket, or sports event, or even turn on the television, and you'll probably see the name *Swisse Wellness*, Australia's most popular vitamin and supplements manufacturer. Its name used to be *Swisse Vitamins*, until, around 2015, it was taken over by listed Hong Kong-based company Biostime International Holdings, and someone had the idea to drop the namesake of its core product and tap into something much bigger. Among the $1.6 billion company's celebrity ambassadors have been Hollywood actress Nicole Kidman and cricketer Ricky Ponting, both of whom have featured on commercials with the tagline, 'You'll feel better on Swisse', despite a federal watchdog finding in 2012 that there was no evidence most people got any benefit from taking many of its products.

Wellness stores today offer body scrubs and facials, and department-store chains now devote entire sections to wellness products. In 2017, Saks Fifth Avenue's flagship store in Manhattan renamed its second floor 'The Wellery'. Covering 1,500 square metres, The Wellery provides exercise classes, brow bars, vegan non-toxic manicures, cellulite treatment, salt-detoxification booths, and, in its clothing range, it stocks golf wear and activewear.

Workplace wellness programs are another of wellness's best-known adaptations today. Half of all US employers with 50 staff or more are estimated to have one in place. But its definition here, too, is largely pared back, often focusing on things such as body-mass indexes, cholesterol checks, blood pressure, and perhaps some yoga, but overlooking many of wellness's core aspects outside of physical health.

John spent 30 years fighting to get Halbert Dunn's ideas out into the world, and now 'there's a wellness centre on every street corner', bearing scant resemblance to its original philosophy. It once frustrated him, seeing 'wellness' being thrown around and used as a marketing buzzword in a cheap bid to garner attention. The last time he typed 'wellness' into Google, the No. 1 hit that came back was some sort of all-natural dog-food brand.

But that's not what upsets him the most about the devolution of the term. John seems much more distressed by another way that wellness has come to be used: the *medicalisation* of wellness; the notion that wellness can be used to *treat* health problems.

'Wellness is about learning and it's about growing,' John explains. 'It's not about fixing things.' Wellness could just as easily be founded in psychology or sociology as it could be in healthcare, he says.

Few cancer specialists dispute the idea that many therapies falling under today's big umbrella of wellness *can* have a positive effect on patients. When used in tandem with chemotherapy, radiation therapy, and surgery, things such as yoga, massage, meditation, acupuncture, aromatherapy, and relaxation techniques constitute what cancer doctors now refer to as 'complementary' therapies. The Cancer Council advises patients that such therapies can help them manage the symptoms of the disease and the side effects of treatment, as well as relieve stress and anxiety. The famous singer, actor, and cancer-awareness advocate Olivia Newton-John, in 2012, permitted Melbourne's Austin Hospital to use her name in its new $189 million cancer wing on two conditions: first, that it incorporate the word *wellness* and, second, that it offer wellness therapies to ease physical, emotional, and spiritual pain. (When, in 2017, Newton-John revealed that her breast cancer had returned, she said she would complete a course of radiation treatment in conjunction with 'natural wellness therapies'.)

Then, however, there are the more extreme, more cultish, and far more disturbing manifestations of wellness theories in cancer treatment: where wellness becomes a synonym for alternative medicine; where it becomes about *curing* the disease. Once confined to the fringes of the wellness movement, the advent of social media has propelled this most controversial aspect into a world of its own. A world of pseudoscience, fad diets, juice cleanses, and miracle cures. A world of popular *wellness warriors*, like Jess Ainscough and her heir apparent, Belle Gibson.

For Ainscough and Gibson, and wellness warriors like them, their interpretation of the word *wellness* goes beyond the down-to-earth values, and attention to mind and body and spirit and environment. Wellness, for them, often means distrusting conventional medicine and believing in unproven treatments such as extreme dieting, colonic irrigation, or high doses of vitamins and antioxidants instead. You might also hear these sorts of people claiming that cancer battles boil down to having the right attitude or willpower to survive. At best, according to experts at the Cancer Council, these theories can be misleading and expensive, and provide false hope. At worst, they encourage vulnerable people to withdraw from treatments that give them the best chance of survival.

'Drugs do not cure cancer,' Ainscough once wrote. 'They just don't. Cancer is nothing more than your body telling you that something has got to give. It is the result of a breakdown in your body's defenses after it has endured years of abuse in the form of a toxic diet, toxic mind and toxic environment. I feel so, so blessed to be wise to these facts.'

When it comes to Ainscough, and the new wave of so-called wellness bloggers who ply their miracle cures online, prominent naturopath Grace Gawler is scathing. 'Sweet-faced, ill-informed young women,' is how she describes them. 'I'm sure — or at least, I hope — they have no idea of the influence and impact they are having on the lives of cancer patients.' When she was a young woman herself, Gawler, too, was a part of the wellness movement, but this was before there was a strong counter-narrative to accepted science, back when it was about 'merging the best of both worlds, complementary and conventional'.

When wellness was born out of the 1970s New Age revolution, and popularised by the likes of John Travis and Don Ardell, it was a 'new path that promised health, wellbeing, longevity, and enlightenment', Gawler explains. By the end of that decade, wellness had taken a noticeable turn. 'Some stayed true to the real pursuit of wellness,' she says, 'but many saw the economic opportunity of blending wellness, treatment, and spirituality and selling it as a cure-all.' In the 1980s, Gawler continues, unsubstantiated stories of miracle cancer healings brought about through diets, meditation, and positive thinking abounded. But it was perhaps not until the advent of the internet that wellness and the treatment of diseases became inextricably bound. 'Access to the internet provided a conveyor belt of opinions, pseudoscience, fake news, and opportunity for anyone to peddle their cyber health-wares. Some had their 15 minutes of fame; some became folk heroes of the online cancer world.'

Gawler is the ex-wife of the controversial Australian cancer guru Ian Gawler, with whom she established an cancer support group in the early 1980s, founded in teachings about nutrition, meditation, and the power of the mind. Ian Gawler claimed to have cured himself of secondary bone cancer in the 1970s, and authored a popular book, *You Can Cure Cancer*. In more recent years, doubts have surrounded whether he ever had advanced cancer at all, with two eminent oncologists suggesting he in fact had tuberculosis. Ian, who still runs the popular natural-healing program he set up with Grace, disputes this hypothesis. Grace now runs an organisation on the Gold Coast offering 'cancer navigation' services to patients.

After four decades working with more than 18,000 cancer patients, Grace Gawler still believes in the benefits of complementary treatments, but is frank in her advice that wellness therapies cannot kill the disease. Grace, who has seen many cancer patients die prematurely because they put their trust in unproven ideas, now describes herself as someone who 'shepherds' patients back to conventional medicine. 'Forty-two years into my career has shown me more misery, pain, and suffering from patients following unproven advice than I could have imagined,' she says. 'In the past, patients turned to alternatives when they had no viable medical options. Today, too many patients turn to alternatives, turning away from viable medical options, based on a whim and an ideology.'

For Gawler, the silver lining of the Belle Gibson saga is that it has helped lift the lid on the darkness that has gripped the wellness industry, which, she says, is 'rotten to the core'. 'It has lost a connection to the very humanistic values that in the beginning, made it so special,' she says. 'For our physical and psychological wellbeing, we need to take a long, hard look at the remedies.'

When the idea of wellness first shot to national attention, and John Travis appeared on the US's *60 Minutes* programme in November 1979, host Dan Rather, sitting across from him, asked a question about wellness that was on a lot of people's minds: Is it meant to be a substitute practice of medicine?

'Absolutely not,' John returned frankly. 'It is an adjunct to, and quite different to, the practise of medicine.'

Until just recently, John had never heard of Belle Gibson. But he has seen plenty of others like her, and seen them come and go: people who claim to be treating their varied diseases with wellness.

'What she was doing is not what wellness is. Wellness is growth, and learning about yourself, and expanding your horizons,' John says, easing back in his deck chair again.

'But I'm afraid a lot of that falls on deaf ears.'

5

FRIENDS IN HIGH PLACES

Less than two weeks after Belle Gibson's app went live, a thrilling email landed in her inbox. It was from an executive at Apple. He was writing to congratulate her on The Whole Pantry's meteoric success, and wanted to fly to Melbourne to meet her. 'When we met,' Gibson wrote in her book, 'he told me that Apple had never seen an app launch in Australia the way mine had.' More than two million apps were available on the Apple Store that year, and Gibson's had been singled out from the crowd. It was the beginning of an exciting partnership that would see her invited to Apple Inc's corporate headquarters in Cupertino, California, to work in secret on the smartwatch prototype.

In a matter of months, the young mum and high-school drop-out from Brisbane had launched a start-up that caught the attention of the world's most valuable company. Gibson had come a long way from Wynnum. A fake story on social media had snowballed into a business that was about to go global. Things were moving very quickly indeed. On Instagram, Gibson was *Instafamous*. Now she was becoming mainstream famous, and wealthier by the day.

There was no better time to pitch a cookbook. On the afternoon of 18 September 2013, Gibson typed out an email to Penguin editor Nicole Abadee, spruiking her app's international triumph and her growing social-media presence. She wrote that she had already been approached by a few other publishing houses, but Penguin was a favourite. Gibson's proposal was heavy on the cancer story. In her pitch, she said she had terminal brain cancer, but had surpassed the expectations of her 'specialists and diagnosis' due to a 'holistic and nutritional approach to wellbeing'.

Just a few weeks later, Gibson had an appointment at the publisher's offices, sitting down face-to-face with Julie Gibbs, the director of Penguin's lifestyle imprint, Lantern. Julie — *Jewels* to her team — is a slimly built woman with a wide smile and auburn hair. She had been with Penguin for more than two decades and, for most of that time, she ran Lantern, which she founded in 2004. Regarded as the queen of lifestyle publishing in Australia, Julie was the woman behind some of the most popular (and expensive) cookbooks ever produced. She had worked with the likes of Maggie Beer, Megan Morton, Lucio Galletto, Kylie Kwong, and Matt Moran, and she curated Stephanie Alexander's iconic two-kilogram culinary volume, *The Cook's Companion*, which, since 1996, has sold half a million copies. Julie worked out of a stylish second-floor office in a building in Surry Hills, Sydney, that was filled with colour and unique pieces of furniture, a bespoke bookshelf, and bold, floral-printed arm chairs. There were flowers in vases, and art on the walls. And books, everywhere. It is clear from their early correspondence that Julie was quite taken by Gibson. After their meeting, Julie sent her newest author a bottle of apple cider vinegar, a popular natural-health tonic purported to be a cure-all. She later sent her more gifts, a bundle of books, and a message on her birthday.

She lavished praise on Gibson over what she described as an 'excellent' book proposal. 'I would so love to work with you to make your first book the very best, most inspiring book it could possibly be,' Julie wrote. 'I have been publishing in the health and wellbeing genre for many years now. Your voice and brand has a unique essence about it and we would undertake to respect, cherish and enhance that essence in the preparation and publishing of *The Whole Pantry* book.' Already, Julie was flagging plans for the book to go global. Importantly, she told Gibson, the book would include a 'substantial introduction' telling 'the key points of your personal health odyssey and the powerful benefits you have had from eating and living the way you do'. Her sales and marketing team were excited, too. They could see it was destined for success. 'I understand and live your values and would relish the chance to help you take them to the widest possible book audience,' Julie told Gibson. Katrina O'Brien, Lantern's publishing manager, emailed Gibson a couple of weeks later, saying that Julie was 'so thrilled' to be publishing her cookbook. 'Welcome to Lantern,' Katrina said. 'I'm sure we'll have a great time working together.'

Gibson and Julie sealed the deal. They agreed that Gibson would deliver between 80 and 90 recipes with the help of a 'home economist' that Penguin would fund to the tune of $15,000. The publisher would also front up $12,500, roughly half the cost, to pay for the photography. Gibson's 250-page health and recipe book would have an emphasis on 'cutting out high allergen foods, gluten and sugar from the diet'. And it would contain 'extra informative text about health and lifestyle tips and suggestions'. The first-time author's advance was hefty. Paid over three instalments, it totalled $132,500. At the top of page five of the contract that Gibson signed on 19 November 2013, the author was required to warrant that no part of the work would be 'a false representation, or misleading or deceptive or likely to mislead or deceive'. Belle Gibson initialled the bottom right-hand corner of the page — as she did on all the other pages of the contract.

Gibson's relationship with Julie and the Lantern team blossomed over the next 12 months. The emails exchanged reveal that the publishing staff were incredibly supportive and caring, and believed in their new star author. And Gibson, for her part, seemed grateful for the opportunity she'd been given. Once, Julie arrived back at her office after a sales conference to find a present from Gibson waiting for her. It was *La Tavola Della Famiglia*, a cookbook about a Melbourne restaurant family, the Bortolottos.

Julie emailed Gibson 'an enormous thank you':

> I can't tell you how special that book is. For several reasons: It is a beautiful book about a wonderful Melbourne restaurant family. When I lived in Melbourne 25 years ago I often used to dine at their St Kilda restaurant Bortolottos with Stephanie Alexander. The photos were taken by the gorgeous Sharyn Cairns and styled by the immensely talented Lee Blaylock. Mostly because you had the big heart to know I would love it and to gift it. Thank you so much.
>
> We are hard at work on your book. Still material being compiled and polished but we will get there! It's going to be wonderful. Hope all is well and that you are happy and stimulated but not too exhausted.
>
> Love Julie

The Whole Pantry, when it was published, was beautiful. It was heavy and full of healthy, do-able, and down-to-earth recipes accompanied by stunning photography showing the texture, colour and depth of food. It featured quinoa tortillas, buckwheat and rosehip bircher, zucchini and chocolate muffins, lentil shepherd's pie, fermented veggies, spiced pumpkin seed brittle, and lemon macadamia tarts with baked peaches. Gracing the thick pages were delicate watercolour illustrations. There was beauty advice, and tips on detoxing, on gut health, on weight loss, and on how to avoid chemicals. It contained a chart with natural medicines and instructions on how to make your own cleaning products. The book, and its *whole life* philosophy, encouraged swapping coffee for herbal tea, meditating, drinking more water, exercising, getting enough sleep, and having a break from technology. The pages were interspersed with a few shots of Gibson and Oli shopping at a farmers' market, and splashing their feet in a river and eating black sesame bliss balls on a picnic rug. There was a 3,000-word precede, *The Story So Far*, a question-and-answer style write-up in which Gibson talked about life *pre-cancer*, and explained why she decided to *heal herself*, how she managed the fear of living with a *terminal illness*, the impact the *disease* had on her life, and her hopes for the future.

The front cover of the book whispered of a *back-to-basics approach to wellness, lifestyle and nutrition*. Of course, Gibson had no expertise in any such area. But that didn't matter. Her credentials were listed in the first words of the very first sentence on the back cover: *Social media sensation*.

It's little wonder that a book about healthy food written by a young, photogenic, cancer-curing mother flew off the shelves, just as Penguin knew it would: the first print run was huge, a staggering 42,000 copies. It was priced at $35. Published in Australia in late October 2014, the book had sold more than 16,000 copies by the end of the year. By then, the plan to take *The Whole Pantry* to the rest of the world was well underway. Julie introduced Gibson to her UK team, which included Lindsey Evans, the cookery publisher for Penguin Random House, based at The Strand, in London. 'I know you two will get on a treat,' Julie said. 'Lindsey has worked with

Jamie Oliver for years and is very experienced at high-profile cookery titles.' Lindsey replied that she was delighted to be publishing *The Whole Pantry* in the UK, and her colleague, Tasmin English, couldn't have been more thrilled to be part of the project. 'Your message is such a vital and inspiring one, there is so much common sense in how you approach nutrition,' she wrote to Gibson. 'It's a delight that we can share your ethos and gorgeous recipes with readers this side of the world too!' Penguin's UK publisher, Michael Joseph, and the American publishing house Simon & Schuster, were to release *The Whole Pantry* cookbook in the northern hemisphere. If questions had not been asked in the media about Gibson's story, her book would have been for sale in bookshops on three continents by mid-2015.

Julie could not have known then what she knows now, but Gibson's book was to be one of her last. In 2013, Penguin was in the midst of a merger with Random House, a merger that would ultimately see Lantern gutted. In mid-2015, just after Gibson had come undone, the newly formed publishing goliath, Penguin Random House, announced it would slash the number of books Lantern printed and that the woman at the helm for more than a decade would, in turn, be leaving the company. Then chief executive Gabrielle Coyne said there simply weren't the commercial returns anymore that there once was in illustrated books.

A few months before Gibson had pitched her book to Julie, the Lantern boss was asked in a media interview what she was most looking forward to. She replied that every year brought new and exciting projects. 'The wonderful thing,' said Julie, 'is that this job is never repetitive or static.' Julie has never spoken publicly about Gibson, but the year she spent working alongside her is one she is not likely to forget.

***

In 2013, Apple awarded Gibson the title of Best New Aussie App, Best Food and Drink App, and runner-up for App of the Year. The Whole Pantry was included in Apple's 'Great Aussie Apps and Games' promotion, included as part of an editor's choice recommendation, and publicised worldwide as a healthy living app. It was translated into French, Spanish, Japanese, and simplified Chinese, and was made available in Australia, the UK, and the US. The app was preinstalled on display iPads featured in Apple stores. Gibson posted a photo of herself peeking over an iPad from inside Apple's New York store on Fifth Avenue, where The Whole Pantry app was being featured.

Apple saw something in Belle Gibson. The star app developer was once quoted as saying, 'As Apple said to me, "Not only did you create a great app, you also created a market for healthy living apps."'

Emails back and forth between senior Apple staff and Gibson speak volumes about how closely she had been embraced by the company. They begin with 'Hello darling one' or 'Lovely' or 'Sweetest', and sign off with kisses. In the acknowledgements section of her book, Gibson specifically singles out three Apple staff. She describes Luke Bevans, the Apple App Store manager for Australia and New Zealand, as her mentor:

> Thank you, for reaching out in our humble beginnings and mentoring me more than you had to. The book wouldn't be without a successful app, and it was you who encouraged me to keep that momentum happening.

Gibson travelled to Japan to meet with Apple executives on the 40th floor of the Mori tower in Roppongi, Tokyo, to discuss a local content and marketing strategy. She toured Apple's headquarters in Cupertino. Three months later, Gibson was back in the US again when The Whole Pantry was announced as one of the few apps handpicked from around the world to be featured as a centrepiece on Apple's new smartwatch. She was the only Australian invited to develop an app for the new device. Her logo, two white leaves on a pale-green background, was all over smartwatch promos, front and centre — twice the size of the Pinterest and Nike logos.

In a recorded interview, Gibson talked about how she was given early access to Apple's smartwatch prototype and the new functions she was developing for the device. 'Apple can surely trust you with a secret. They gave you access, how long ago?' she was asked.

'Three-and-a-half weeks ago,' she replied, 'and we're the only team from Australia, so we're feeling very proud and honoured. If there was any company that we were going to jump for, it was going to be Apple because they've supported us for so long.'

Asked about how her health was then, Gibson paused for a couple of seconds and considered her answer. 'I … It's funny that I'm here,' she began. 'All of my friends and family said, "Belle, you can't go." Six weeks ago, um, I was re-diagnosed with multiple cancers, um, but I'm feeling on top of the world.'

Gibson was beaming. Photos from the event show her grinning widely and wearing a long-sleeved, white fitted shirt, with an Apple swipe card hanging around her neck. She's standing in a room full of people, in front of a large white screen with the iconic Apple logo, emblazoned in black, behind her. While in the US, Gibson went online and posted an inspirational quote from Apple founder Steve Jobs: 'If you do something and it turns out pretty good, then you should go do something else wonderful, not dwell on it for too long. Just figure out what's next – Steve.' The post was 'liked' by thousands of her followers.

Back in Australia, Gibson was asked to appear on a panel at an Apple retail store event in Sydney to discuss her success building

The Whole Pantry. The invitation plugged Gibson's own tagline: 'The Whole Pantry is the first app of its kind, combining inspiring wholefood recipes with lifestyle and wellness guides.' It was a warm summer evening when Gibson appeared on stage in Apple's George Street store. She sat next to a staff member wearing the company's trademark blue T-shirt. Dressed all in black, Gibson spoke to her captivated audience of young people, and fielded questions from the crowd. 'It was quite busy,' said Sydney yoga teacher Roshini McCartin. 'People had to stand.'

Roshini became a big fan of Gibson's after coming across her on Instagram. She had the app on her phone, and later bought the book. The Apple event was promoting app-building, holding Gibson up as a success story. But Roshini wasn't there to learn about building an app. She was there to see Gibson in the flesh. She said Gibson had a young, girl-next-door kind of feel about her. She wasn't airbrushed. She was raw and relatable. 'I remember her sharing a little bit about her story, her cancer, her child, the success of her app,' Roshini recalls. 'I walked away super inspired. I thought, *Wow, anything is possible*. I believed every single word she said, and I'm quite a good judge of character.'

In her book, Gibson thanks Bree McKenzie, an Apple events and marketing manager, 'for creating a dream with me in your Sydney Apple Store — a moment that still blows me away, and one that wouldn't have happened if you didn't believe in the TWP message or hard work.'

Apple's public relations and marketing staff introduced Gibson to the media so that she could promote her app. 'Once Apple saw the app,' the company would later tell the courts, 'it was decided that Apple Australia would make an effort to introduce the developer (Annabelle Gibson) to the Australian media.'

An Apple executive once emailed Gibson to tell her that the

app store URL featuring her book and app had gone live. Apple's marketing team in Cupertino contacted Gibson asking for exclusive promo art so her app could be featured on the App Store's Facebook and Twitter pages. The company's publicity arm kept her in mind for developer profiles that they could put forward to the media for 'wellness-related stories'. In one pitch to a Sydney newspaper, Gibson was included as a part of a package on *Female developers who are changing the world one app at a time!* 'A single mum who was diagnosed with cancer, Belle turned to whole food cooking and eating,' the promo from Apple began. 'She wanted to share what she learnt but didn't want to use a website or blog. Belle decided she wanted to build an app for iPhone and iPad. She spent hours learning how to "code" and took a very active role in the process to ensure every last detail was to her spec.'

Jesse James, Apple's Australian PR manager, became very close with Gibson. She typed out a message on her iPhone 5s saying she was more than happy to help Gibson workshop a media plan so her message didn't get lost. 'I agree you should not do any more interviews until you work out exactly what you want your story to be — being a female app developer who's innovating like crazy is getting lost,' Jesse wrote.

TC Chan, another Apple employee, was also known to have a close relationship with Gibson. Some described him as her 'handler' in Australia for Apple Inc. In her tribute to TC in the back of her book, Gibson thanked him for encouraging and helping her: 'Because you're the only one who understands the fragmented, colliding universe with me.' TC is a middle-aged man from Sydney. One former friend of Gibson's described her relationship with TC as 'extremely close' and 'very odd'. 'They would sit there holding hands,' he said. 'But you've got to remember, people were just so emotionally involved with her story at the time.'

Cosmopolitan magazine nominated Gibson for an award, and invited her to a photoshoot at the Skyline drive-in theatre in Blacktown, western Sydney. She posed next to singer-songwriter Dami Im in the 1950s diner-style shoot. Staff remember an Apple representative, believed to be TC, watching on from the sidelines. 'He was rapped [sic] with her,' one said. 'He was talking about how exciting the [Apple] watch was going to be and the fact that there were very, very few apps that were going to be built into the watch and TWP was one of them.'

Gibson took to social media again and again to praise her 'gorgeous team at Apple who helped this dream come alive,' singling out Luke Bevans and TC Chan.

Gibson was once asked to name her biggest influence on her 'health journey'. 'Steve Jobs,' she replied. 'It's bizarre, I know, but I really do admire his vision and how much he fought for what he believed in.'

It certainly was bizarre. The founder of Apple died from pancreatic cancer in 2011, after delaying surgery for nine months and opting instead to go down an alternative-treatment route, using fruit juices, dietary supplements, and acupuncture to try to fight the disease. After his death, his biographer, Walter Isaacson, a former *TIME* magazine editor, said Jobs regretted his decision not to use conventional medicine sooner, and believed he had made a mistake. 'We talked about this a lot,' Isaacson said. 'He wanted to talk about it, how he regretted it. I think he felt he should have been operated on sooner.'

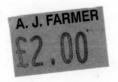

6

THE BEST YEAR

'It's time to have the most inspiring and empowering people that have encouraged this journey in a room together,' Gibson wrote in the online invite to the launch party of The Whole Pantry app. It was typed on a white background with splashes of green watercolour paint around the edges, and told guests about the charities the event would be supporting: asylum-seekers, birthing kits for women in developing countries, school-building in Sierra Leone, and the family of a five-year-old Melbourne boy with terminal brain cancer. Gibson asked her guests to come to the big night, on 6 December 2013, with money in their pockets to donate to the worthy causes.

The call-out went far and wide. It was emailed to everyone on Gibson's mailing list. But she made it clear that while she was soliciting donations to support people in need, not everyone was invited to the *actual* launch party: 'We wish you could all be part of our world-changing events but unfortunately we haven't yet found a room big enough, so instead we are selling virtual tickets

THE BEST YEAR 57

with proceeds going to the four charities.' Virtual tickets, as she called them, were sold online through Eventbrite. People could purchase anything from a general admission ticket for $20 to a VIP reserved ticket for $100. Or they could name their price. This way, Gibson said, people could still be part of the event, feel part of her community, even though they couldn't come.

The app launch and fundraiser night was held at The White House, an ornate St Kilda mansion on Princes Street, built in the mid-1800s for Victoria's crown solicitor. It's now the home base to Small Giants, an organisation that works with businesses which have a social or environmentally sustainable streak, such as TOM Organic, which sells a range of certified organic tampons and pads, and independent magazine *Dumbo Feather*. Gibson, who had struck up a friendship with TOM Organic founder Aimee Marks, had managed to get a cut-price 'friends and family' rate to hire the ballroom for two hours.

Guests started arriving just after 6.30 pm. It was a Friday at the start of summer. The clocks had gone forward, and the sun was staying out for longer. It was a warm night, and natural light lit up the stately room. A large table stretching down the centre was draped in Bonnie and Neil tablecloths, made from oat linen, and screen printed in floral patterns of turquoise green and purple-blue. They were laden with food made from the recipes featured in Gibson's app.

Gibson's closest friends were in the kitchen preparing the food. There were canapés and drinks. A dark cake was topped with pomegranate, strawberries, and raspberries. Chocolate mousse was sprinkled with little purple-and-yellow edible flowers, served in wine glasses, out of a rustic wooden crate. And there were bunches of beautiful flowers everywhere. Guests filled a glass bowl with cash and coins, and wrote IOUs on pieces of paper nominating their intended charities. They remember an intimate gathering — a few dozen people were there — and they felt honoured to be on the exclusive invite list.

Gibson was heavily made-up, and looked dazzling. Her long hair was styled, and she wore a halter dress by Australian designer Scanlan & Theodore that was white, backless, and flared above the knee. Gibson mingled with guests under the antique chandelier and around the black grand piano. She looked the picture of health.

Gibson was always very particular about whom she connected with. She associated herself with people who were making waves: other health gurus, entrepreneurs, people with their own online followings. Gibson had been embraced by the wellness community, yoga teachers and naturopaths, and people selling raw food and organic tea. Among her friends, she listed soap actress-turned-life coach Melissa Ambrosini, and the well-known nutritionist and prolific author Lola Berry. Others included Sarah Ranawake, a former features director at *Cleo* magazine and the founder of online fashion and health magazine *Sporteluxe*; vegan cook and author Kate Bradley; and the late Polly Noble, an English health coach who died from cervical cancer in 2014. She ranked among her friends small-business owners such as Nat Warner, from cold-pressed Prahran juice company Greene Street Juice Co., and Georgie Castle, who founded vegan chocolate company Citizen Cacao, and Colly Galbiati, the owner of Australian food company Soma Organics. As a mentor, she singled out Charlie Goldsmith, a PR expert and self-proclaimed 'energy healer' who is set to star in a US television series where he attempts to cure the sick.

On the night of the app launch, businesswomen Bree Johnson and Erika Geraerts, co-founders of the $20 million-a-year skincare line Frank Body, attended. So, too, did Lisa Hamilton, a fashion blogger with 350,000 Instagram followers who launched the website

SeeWantShop. Diamond Rozakeas, one of the owners of a string of Melbourne's most successful cafés, including Top Paddock in Richmond and The Kettle Black in South Melbourne, came with her partner. Melbourne wellness coaches and business owners and social-media influencers posed arm-in-arm around Gibson.

'She knew the who's who of Melbourne,' said one business owner. 'Lots of entrepreneurs and go-getters. They were always in the room, always backing her.'

'The attraction was her interesting medical condition,' said attendee Kenneth Meow, a Melbourne foodie, whose Instagram account is dedicated to promoting the local café scene. He was interested in knowing more about the young cancer-fighting mother who was using the profit from her app to help others.

As always, Gibson made a heart-warming speech. Standing in front of a decorative fireplace with wild flowers on the mantle behind her, she spoke about her cancer diagnosis, her 'journey to wholefoods,' her vision for a healthier world. Her guests cried. Yoga teacher Monica Aurora remembers the feeling in the room. Here was this young woman who had defied the odds to overcome certain death, was living for her son, and she was positively thriving. 'There were people up the front fully crying and donating all this money,' Monica recalls. 'It was a big thing, a big show.' Kate Toholka was moved, too. She came to the event after meeting Gibson on Instagram some months earlier. Kate was blogging a lot at the time; it had been an outlet for her after she moved from the city to the Surf Coast. Gibson's speech inspired her to dedicate a blog entry the following week about the young starlet's 'beautiful journey from inspired idea to kicking arse!' And before she left, like just about everyone else, she dropped some money into the glass bowl.

***

The year 2014 was Belle Gibson's best. She had been anointed by Apple, and she had a book deal in the bag. The cheques kept coming, and Gibson wasted no time trading up. She bought a brand-new BMW X3, and had her teeth cosmetically straightened. She started dressing for her new life as a wellness star. Her style was voguish, with a hint of hippie: the ring in her nose and the black-and-gold Alexander Wang handbag over her shoulder; the yin yang tattoo on her forearm above a Georg Jensen watch. Gibson looked fashionable yet wholesome; she wore oversized rings and sunglasses, and shopped at local organic green grocers.

Gibson, the 'cancer survivor' and wellness guru, was cashing in. At the height of her fame, she moved into a residence more befitting of a young internet entrepreneur — a $1 million beachside townhouse she rented for more than $1,000 a week just off the picture-book Elwood Esplanade. The double-storey Wilton Grove apartment is 200 metres from the water. Its real-estate listing boasts 'cutting-edge design, the highest quality finishes, [and a] commanding street presence'. It has three bedrooms, three bathrooms, a large wine cellar, Italian tiling and hardwood floors, video intercom, a fireplace, private decking, and an open-plan kitchen with Miele appliances. 'Exquisite in every way,' reads the ad, 'luxurious and beautifully appointed'.

Gibson furnished the apartment stylishly: a grey designer couch; retro laminate dining table and Danish-style wooden chairs; unique prints and a black-and-white photo of Bob Dylan sitting at a piano; piles and piles of cookbooks, stacked perfectly for a #shelfie Instagram post.

In an unusual twist, the modern, cube-style property that Gibson and her family moved into is owned by the Melbourne boss of Google, Sean McDonell, and his wife, Kate. Gibson rented the property through an estate agent while McDonell was working for the internet giant in Sydney. Google refused to comment when we asked if McDonell and Gibson had any professional relationship.

Gibson had a good life in the inner south-eastern suburbs of Melbourne, one of the most affluent parts of the city. She would shop and dine out with friends in Prahran, Windsor, and South Yarra, get her nails done in Balaclava, visit a massage therapist in St Kilda. She frequented upscale cafés and restaurants, and cute little stationery stores. Her local village grocer in Elwood was a favourite.

Everyone who met Gibson during this time described her as pleasant, friendly, polite, and generous. 'She was lovely, really lovely,' said one. Some people said that she sometimes seemed 'vague' or a bit 'spacey', but they just put that down to her medical condition. Gibson supported local artists and independent craft shops. She'd go to Red Stitch Actors Theatre in St Kilda East, and visit the Arts Centre. She liked upmarket homewares stores in South Melbourne, and an artisan coffee shop in Albert Park. Sometimes she'd cross town to Northcote to go to the Terra Madre organic shop and wellness clinic. Gibson visited bookstores and markets, and bought things like *Good Brew Kombucha* and $48-a-box recycled toilet paper. Her new car cost $1187.62 a month, and she'd spend $350 at an Armadale hair salon.

She went away on location, with her team, to the charming rural town of Daylesford, outside Melbourne, at the foothills of the Great Dividing Range, to shoot the images for her cookbook. To unwind, she took an ocean cruise to the Pacific Islands. 'She was clearly coming from a space of, *I'm successful, I've made so much money from the app*,' said a former friend. 'We thought she was all that.'

Gibson wanted to lose four kilograms. She bought the Kayla Itsines' Bikini Body Bundle, and started seeing Lachlan Clarke, a high-profile personal trainer, once dubbed 'Melbourne's model trainer', who had a reputation for sculpting a healthy, toned, and lean physique. His business was called Body Psyche, and he charged $99 an hour for tailored one-on-one sessions in his studio in Abbotsford. Lachlan said one of his clients, a fashion model from the Chadwicks modelling agency, had referred Gibson to him, and he did 10 sessions with her.

Lachlan is very tanned and absurdly trim. He wears low-slung T-shirts and has a large Adam's apple. His hair is coiffed, his stubble thick and short. He talks fast, but when it comes to health and fitness, he is a qualified exercise coach who knows what he's talking about, and, after a little while, Gibson began to seek out and to value his opinions. They would often send each other links to nutrition articles and workout videos. Outside their sessions in the studio, the pair caught up a couple of times, and developed a friendship. Of all the people in Gibson's circle, everyone named and acknowledged in the back of her book, Lachlan appears to have been the only one in these early years, when her star was rising, who pulled her up. Everyone else, it seems, showered her in unconditional praise. He felt obliged to say something: about her extreme dieting advice that was encouraging people to cut out entire food groups; the things she was saying about nutrition and the human body that simply weren't true. 'I call a spade a spade,' said Lachlan, 'and was incredibly blunt with her.'

One morning, they met up at the Weylandts Kitchen, a café near Lachlan's studio. Lachlan hadn't seen Gibson for some time, not since she had returned from her trip with Apple to the US. He had been reading much of her writing, and had typed out an entire page of notes. 'She was getting into the dangerous world of dictating advice to people, and people were listening,' he said, 'but she was someone who never grasped the fundamentals … she didn't know what she was talking about.' Lachlan chose a table at the café that would be the furthest away from prying eyes. He was ready to unload on her.

Gibson sat down and ordered a peppermint tea. 'A lot of what she was claiming was just fucking irresponsible. I pulled her up on some of the things she was saying, like saying coconut oil hydrates connective tissue … "You can't say that", I told her. "It's bullshit."'

Gibson became defensive, and said, 'Well, that's just your opinion,' recalls Lachlan. 'She didn't care how valid her information was.' Lachlan was concerned about the trend he was seeing on social media where people were increasingly turning to Instagram celebrities for health and fitness advice, instead of seeking out professionals. But it was too late. Gibson was already a star on Instagram, and she was fast becoming well known in wellness circles.

Gibson was selected to go on a creative retreat to Bali with a group of about two dozen women, including her good friend and one of the former directors of Kinfolk café, Bec Villanti. The retreat was run by singer-songwriter Clare Bowditch's organisation, Big Hearted Business. Those who were chosen spent a week in Ubud with Clare and her closest friends singing and dancing and meditating, and taking part in personal-development classes. They stayed in beautiful villas with private lagoon-shaped pools, shaded by palm trees and overlooking rice fields. Gibson booked a place for her family so they could all be together, and also travelled to Seminyak on the holiday. There's a warm, smiling photo of Gibson standing cheek-to-cheek with Clare and Melbourne life coach Julie Parker. In another close-up photo of Julie and Gibson, taken in Bali, Julie talks about how blessed she feels to be on the retreat and how honoured she is to spend more time with 'one of the most inspirational women I know'.

'This lady is changing the world with her grace, beauty and courage,' she wrote. 'She is Big Hearted Business personified.' Julie is the founder of the Beautiful You Coaching Academy and the author of *Inspired Coach* magazine. Clare Bowditch has graced the front page, and the first-ever edition featured bestselling self-help author Melissa Ambrosini on the cover. Among the glowing endorsements of Gibson's book and app to flood social-media pages for the best part of 18 months were those from Ambrosini, who was also a close friend of 'Wellness Warrior' Jess Ainscough. Ambrosini lives in Bondi Beach. She became close with Gibson as her star was rising, and they caught up when she was in Melbourne. Ambrosini had her tips about de-stressing published on The Whole Pantry app. 'Soulsister' is how she referred to Gibson. 'I'm so grateful to be part of such an amazing product and even more grateful to call Belle my sister,' she once wrote. 'What an inspiration.'

Nutritionist Lola Berry met Gibson at an event in Melbourne in 2013, at the beginning of the rise of health influences on social media. The two quickly became close. Like everyone else, Lola was moved by Gibson's story of survival. She wanted to help her. Sometimes Lola drove Gibson around because she didn't yet have her licence. Lola was also named as a contributor to a guide on The Whole Pantry app, called 'being in the moment with food'. Colly Galbiati, the owner of Australian food company Soma Organics, once posted a photo with the two authors at a Prahran café, describing Gibson as an incredible woman making a difference in the world.

Welltodo, a London-based consultancy firm that advises businesses in the wellness industry, said of Gibson: 'This woman is incredible. She is a game changer and a complete hero. Her story speaks for itself. Follow her, be inspired by her, pray for her.'

Health-food shops, fashion labels, skincare brands, homewares stores, chefs, bloggers, personal trainers, yoga instructors, and photographers posted about the 'amazing', 'inspiring', 'authentic' @healing_belle. *InStyle Australia* promoted her 'healthy' Instagram feed. Cold-pressed juice company The Seed Bali celebrated Gibson on International Women's Day for the 'goodness you offer to the world'. Her fans compared her to Gandhi. One said her book was an 'eye opener', praised Gibson's wisdom, and said she'd follow her footsteps to boost her own health and wellbeing.

In 2014, *Cosmopolitan* magazine awarded Gibson its *Fun, Fearless Female Award* in the social-media category. Gibson flew in from Melbourne for the star-studded event, held during the day at Otto Ristorante in Sydney. The Italian restaurant is on the wharf at Woolloomooloo. Gibson arrived late, just as dessert was being served, and took her seat. She sipped sparkling water, but didn't touch the food. Then her name was called. She'd won by a landslide, receiving thousands more votes than the other women in her category. Dressed in a white, loose-fitting top and watermelon-coloured shorts, the 5 foot 5 inch blonde nervously took the podium to accept her award in front of about 100 people, including American actress Tara Reid and Australian model Jesinta Campbell. Watching on were the winners in the other categories, including TV personalities Lisa Wilkinson and Samantha Armytage, actress Demi Harman, singer Dami Im, and snowboarder Torah Bright. Gibson gave a heartfelt speech about her son, Oli, her community — the followers on Instagram — and the legacy she would leave them. 'It was really emotional,' said a former *Cosmopolitan* staffer. 'I remember Belle wasn't crying, but pretty much everyone else was. We were celebrating women, we had all these amazing women in the room, and there pretty much wasn't a dry eye in the house.'

Belle Gibson, apparently dying, had blossomed. She had quickly become an in-demand keynote speaker, sharing the stage with other young business owners and wellness entrepreneurs. She wasn't a natural public speaker, but it worked for her. Her story was incredibly moving. She always held the room.

Gibson appeared the perfect fit for an all-female networking event called Fierce Women, which raises money for cancer research. The exclusive $100-a-head dinner at Rokeby Studios in Collingwood was promoted as a night to inspire. Along with Gibson, TOM Organic founder Aimee Marks, and Emma Seibold, who started Barre Body yoga studios, were asked to speak. The MC on the night was TV personality Gorgi Coghlan, and there was an intimate performance by Aria-award-winning singer Megan Washington.

The organisers of Fierce Women were Melbourne friends Karla Dawes and Cara Norden, who worked in events and PR. Both women had been touched by cancer, and started the event in 2012 to raise money for the Cancer Council of Victoria. The idea was to host a beautiful, highly curated evening for women, run by women, with all proceeds donated to charity. They're proud to have showcased the stories of many inspirational women and to have raised more than $50,000 for cancer research over the past five years. Karla and Cara didn't know Gibson personally, but asked her to speak because she was 'seen as an inspiration in the wellness space' and was proving herself as a successful entrepreneur. Like the other 130 women there that night, they had no reason to doubt her story.

After Gibson's speech, everyone gave her a standing ovation. 'I was hysterical when she was talking,' said one business owner. 'The way she spoke, it was so devastating.'

'The whole room was crying,' said another. 'She had us all convinced.'

Gibson had grand plans to expand her business. The Whole Pantry was to morph into The Whole *Life*. The new domain name was registered, and Gibson placed a job advertisement to recruit a digital designer. 'We are looking at adding complementary apps to the family, including others outside of our current category that still support the interests of our current users,' she wrote. Gibson said a second book was in the works 'with a focus on community, the revolution of living The Whole Life and stories [from] within the community.'

According to her glossy three-page proposal for The Whole Life, she was going to create a social enterprise: a space for entrepreneurs to meet, collaborate, and host events. Gibson wrote that 'all profits' were given away to those in need. 'We really care about the earth, its communities and their local environments,' Gibson said. 'App sales are donated to rotating charities and organisations that support the health and wellbeing of those globally, protecting and conserving the environment and giving education to those who otherwise don't have the opportunity.'

She took on an assistant and hired a consultant to negotiate office space for her in South Melbourne. Gibson chose a charming Victorian terrace on Cecil Street. The double-storey building has seven offices, a boardroom, bay windows, and marble fireplaces. Gibson signed a three-year, $70,000-a-year lease. She developed a 'furniture proposal' that she had her volunteers pitch to high-end designers in an effort to fit out her new offices for free.

Gibson had plans for a standalone kids app. And she set her sights on the Royal Children's Hospital. She had a proposal to lease space in its new commercial precinct to set up a 'The Whole Pantry kitchen and kiosk'. The North Melbourne hospital's $1 billion re-development includes shops, restaurants, and a hotel for families of sick children. Before it opened, Gibson toured the site, wearing a hardhat and high-vis vest, pointing out potential opportunities for her shop. According to her submission to the hospital's board, her vision was to provide 'nurturing wholefoods for those in need most'. In the submission, which is under her company name, Gibson writes about her commitment to low-waste packaging, and her support for farmers by using seasonal and local ingredients. Gibson's vision included a herbal-tea menu, cold-pressed juices, healthy soups, and chocolate. 'Keeping in line with our successful core food principles on The Whole Pantry app, we continue to offer recipes and meals which are low-inflammatory and free from gluten, GMOs [genetically modified organisms], refined sugar, corn … soy, peanuts etc,' she wrote. According to one source familiar with the proposal, Gibson's sights were set on the soon-to-be-built hotel. 'She wanted a retail space in there to do healthy meals for the parents of sick kids and tap into the hotel, do in-room dining and a kiosk type thing' they said.

Gibson's 2014 proposal included a copy of her CV, in which she described herself as a 'mama, writer, gamechanger'. What is noticeable about this document is what was missing. Gibson was applying for retail space in one of Australia's best-known hospitals, yet she provided little quantifiable information about herself or her business. The document was also full of fabrications. In it, Gibson wrote that 'all profits' from app sales 'go directly back' to the community, donated to rotating charities supporting health, education, and environmental conservation. 'We feel that everyone already part of The Whole Pantry community … are in a privileged position to be able to access their whole life. We feel it's important that part of their spending goes to help those who aren't as privileged.'

Fairbank Grange Property had a deal with the hospital to sublet space in the new development to retailers. Hayden Warszewski, who took applications from retailers vying for space to the hospital, said Gibson's representative called him to talk about her opening a shop there in mid-2014. 'He contacted me and said there's this amazing woman, blah, blah, blah,' Warszewski recalls. 'I put it to the hospital, but it didn't really go much further.'

It is understood the proposal was rejected because of Gibson's support for unproven treatments and her history of making non-evidenced-based medical claims. 'The board's approach is to be very cautious around what kind of retail we promote in the hospital,' one source said, 'and especially cautious if there are any health claims being made.'

Another source said the hospital wouldn't have even given Gibson's proposal serious consideration. 'The position was that [retailers] had to be ethically right, in the same way that we wouldn't have someone in there selling alcohol or tobacco.'

Gibson was wearing a black jacket badged with WWDC, the acronym used by Apple for its yearly Worldwide Developers Conference. Apple selected her to attend the event in June 2014, in San Francisco. She told an interviewer there about her illness and the impetus for building an app. 'I had gone through lots of adversity,' she said, in front of a vegetable display at the Whole Foods Market on 4th Street, just a couple of blocks from the Moscone Center, where the event was being held. 'I still have the cancer, but I'm doing really well, considering.'

The trip wasn't all business. Gibson spent the rest of the month in the US, checking into four- and five-star hotels. She toured West Hollywood and Santa Monica and Venice, and shopped at Trader Joe's and Wholefoods. Then she travelled over to New York, and stayed at the four-star Park Central Hotel. While she was there, Penguin deposited in her bank account the first of three $44,000 instalments for the book advance. A few days later, she spent more than $2,500 at Michael F & Co Inc, a Manhattan jeweller on West 47th Street. Then she went to the IRO New York clothes store, and spent another $500.

In New York City, acai bowl-enthusiast Ksenia Avdulova, the founder of popular website Breakfast Criminals, said she was honoured to meet Gibson while she was in town. She told her legion of online fans about the 'incredibly authentic, driven, beautiful, larger than life' Australian woman with whom she shared a superfoods breakfast at a hotel. 'Belle is one of the most amazing people I've met in this lifetime,' she wrote on her website — in a post that has since been deleted.

Another person who promoted Gibson's app was American wellness blogger Jordan Younger. Jordan is about the same age as Gibson, and she exploded online about the same time. On her blog, *The Blonde Vegan*, Jordan wrote about her vegan diet and healthy lifestyle, and before long she had 70,000 followers. Jordan first met Gibson in New York, and they became fast friends. 'Actually, more than fast friends — we connected on a level of practically soul sisterness that would be hard for me to capture in words,' Jordan told her followers.

Jordan said they held hands and cried together while talking about Gibson's fear of dying from cancer. And that Gibson told her that 100 per cent of sales from The Whole Pantry app and book were donated to charity. Jordan confided in Gibson during that first meeting that she had decided to dump veganism for health reasons, but she didn't yet know how to tell her followers. She was concerned about what it would mean for her future. She said Gibson offered a shoulder to cry on, and then gave her valuable business advice: change the name of her business immediately. Two days later, Jordan went public with the news at an event in New York. Gibson was there, she said, standing at the back of the room, quietly supporting her. Jordan's transition away from veganism earned her a book deal, *Breaking Vegan*, and she is still hugely popular. Her website is now called The Balanced Blonde, and her business has grown into an empire that includes publishing, an app, podcasts, a clothing line, and a range of cleanses.

Jordan remembers the excitement around Gibson in 2014. On the night she went public, she introduced Gibson to her friends in the wellness industry, who were all eager to meet her. 'She was a *huge* inspiration to all of us — a celebrity in the wellness world and a physical embodiment of strength and success in the face of great adversity.'

In the last week of June, Gibson booked a flight with Qantas out of Los Angeles and headed home. Some people quietly expressed wonderment that Gibson, apparently so deathly sick, appeared to be so healthy. She travelled extensively in 2014 — multiple trips to Sydney, Adelaide, Bali, Tokyo, Los Angeles, New York — and yet no one questioned her diagnosis in the early days. Some said later that they had asked themselves about her commitment to her family, to her little boy, about why she would leave him while on round-the-world jaunts while seemingly on the brink of death. But none said anything about that then. 'I didn't question whether she was genuine or not,' said one former friend. 'I just thought, *Where are your priorities: do you want fame and fortune before you die or do you want time with your kid.* [Then I would] just think, *My God, how could you even think that?*

Belle Gibson's cancer story had been in circulation for half a decade. She marked the occasion with a post on Instagram. 'Wow. Holy sh*t,' Gibson wrote:

> Just when I thought this month couldn't get any BIGGER I woke up on my way back home to Australia celebrating with the sunrise over the Pacific. Five years ago today, I was sitting alone in front of a man who was about to tell me I was dying of malignant brain cancer with just six weeks to live. I cared as little as he did and waited the days out. Fast forward soon after, I started a brief relationship with conventional treatment which saw me regress quicker than

imaginable and led me down the life-changing path I'm on today.
It's a surreal morning for me, amongst jet lag, a phenomenal month
in HK and the USA with my community, Apple and my publishers.
I feel so blessed to have seen an opportunity to take control of my
life and health, to be here today, to have the beautiful son I was told
would never happen and be changing the world with each of you
every single day.

Gibson, for a while, was untouchable. And so she went on, tapping
away on her phone, with messages about cancer and medicine and
nutrition echoing far beyond the suburbs of Melbourne, and into
bedrooms and workplaces and oncology wards around the world.

7

NO SUCH THING AS SUPERFOOD

On 4 June 2015, a nutritional scientist named Tim Crowe sat down at his desk, turned on the computer monitor, and quickly got to work on what would become his most popular blog post ever. It was on a subject he had been musing about for quite some time, unsure whether or not he should write it.

Broccoli is bad for you, he eventually keyed into the headline field. *Really toxic bad.* And then he started typing, beginning by stating that broccoli is loaded with goitrogens.

'Goitrogens,' he explained, 'are chemicals that suppress the function of the thyroid gland by interfering with iodine uptake, a key mineral needed to make thyroid hormones. This blocking of iodine uptake causes the thyroid gland to enlarge.'

He went on to explain that broccoli contains particular goitrogenic chemicals called 'thiocyanates'. Eating thiocyanates has the potential to cause 'hypothyroidism,' he said, and that has the potential to cause symptoms such as weight gain, fatigue, depression, hair loss, muscle aches — and so the troubling list went on.

Tim Crowe is a career academic and dietitian, with a PhD and a good reputation. He is lean and clean-shaven, and has thin, dark hair. In his early 40s, he had been 'living and breathing' nutrition for 16 years. His website, *Thinking Nutrition*, launched in 2012, was well regarded in the field as a source of compelling and credible commentary on issues from heart health to weight management, from diabetes to fad diets. It had earned a decent readership by now. But nothing quite like this.

The broccoli post blew up beyond all his expectations. Within days, it had received more than 200,000 clicks (the kind of traffic usually reserved for big mainstream news websites) and was shared on social media more than 10,000 times, far surpassing any article he had published before.

Readers' comments flooded in. It was, after all, a most controversial argument: that what we thought to be one of the healthiest vegetables on the planet could in fact be 'pushing you ever faster to an early grave'.

Some responded out of shock or out of genuine concern.

'What about if young children eat a lot of it?' asked an anxious person called Adam. 'Broccoli is the only veg my 3-year-old will eat so we try to give her some, every other meal time. Could this be bad for her, as she is only a toddler?'

Others blasted the author. 'Whatever!!! Broccoli is a good veggie!!!' another said. 'I don't believe this article!'

Fortunately, many were able to look beyond the startling headline, and had seen Tim's disclaimer. Yes, the science quoted in the article is factual, but no, everything you've been told since childhood about the wholesome green vegetable has not been a barefaced lie. There was no cause for alarm. Broccoli is not bad for you: it is one of the healthiest things you can eat.

Vegetables such as broccoli, spinach, kale, and cauliflower *can* decrease iodine uptake, because they contain goitrogens, but studies suggest you would need to eat about 194 micromoles (25 mg) of goitrogens daily for them to have any effect. To put this in context, that's about two kilograms of broccoli a day.

This was Tim's attempt at making a point — a point about the dangerous intersection of nutrition and the internet. Where grains, soy, gluten, and sugar are regularly condemned as being 'toxic'. As are eggs, coffee, and salt, depending on the day.

Many months later, sitting in an arcade café in Melbourne, Tim orders a coffee. A flat white. With regular milk. Full of lactose. He says that while some people have intolerances to certain products, as a society we are becoming needlessly fearful of many foods. This, he believes, is in a large part because you can build a case for just about anything being bad, by selectively quoting scientific research and blowing it out of context.

And for the same reason, you can build a case for any product you want to market and sell as being good. 'Superfoods', even. Whole industries have flourished around acai, aloe vera, flaxseed, chia seed, and coconut oil. In recent years, farmers around the world have ripped up long-standing vegetable crops to plant millions of kale seeds instead. The Western world has been accused of starving the poor people of Peru and Bolivia out of quinoa, as the cost of the food that has been their staple for thousands of years is driven up by international demand. Goji berries, the first so-called superfood, are still marketed with unsubstantiated claims that a Chinese man who ate handfuls of the berries every day lived to be 256 years old (from 1677 to 1933, apparently).

'They are berries,' says Tim. 'Like *any other berries*. There is a whole myth-creating industry around food, and it works well.'

Glancing around him, Tim turns his attention to one of the latest dietary crazes. The café we are in is one of the many new 'pressed-

2017

juice' shops that have sprung up around the world. This one sells five-day juice-cleanse packages, for $319, promoting everything from a collagen boost to better-oxygenated blood. A few kilometres away, one of its competitor's juice stores has a $67-a-day cleanse for people who are overweight, moody, or want to 'reset the body and mind'.

'People are claiming this gives you energy and makes you lose weight, and here's some dodgy research to support it,' Tim says, resting his coffee cup back down on the table. 'If you're selling dishwashing liquids that's OK, but with nutrition it's dangerous.'

The biggest weakness in the science of nutrition — the unfortunate thing that makes it susceptible to falsehoods, fad diets, and baseless advice — is the lack of rock-solid evidence to base it on. In order to test out hypotheses about what's healthy and what's not in any definitive way, investigative scientists have to carry out rigorous, long-term experiments. The gold standard of these experiments is called the 'randomised controlled trial', and the findings it reaches are the most irrefutable. When it's done using lab rats, it's pretty straightforward. You take two groups of identically bred rats, feed one group diet A (a special diet), and put the other on diet B (a standard diet), and then track their progress to see what happens over their lifespan, which is usually only a year or two.

Humans, however, are not lab rats, and cannot be treated the same. The fact that we can't be force-fed potentially dangerous diets for years at a time in order to test them is undoubtedly a good thing for humans, but a bad thing for the science of nutrition. A set of hugely controversial experiments carried out on patients at a mental hospital in Sweden in the 1940s, called the Vipeholm experiments, for example, taught us much of what we know about dental health. Hundreds of patients there were used as the subjects in large-scale trials in which they were fed copious amounts of sugar, toffee, and various sweets to examine whether sugar-rich diets caused tooth decay. Many of the patients had their teeth completely ruined by the experiments, which were a major violation of medical ethics, but, scientifically speaking, were a massive success.

In today's world, where scientists cannot simply conscript large groups of humans to test out the effects of various diets, controlled trials in nutrition are extremely difficult and expensive to do, and the results they reach are regularly disappointing.

Diet hypotheses are essentially about what will improve or impair our prospects of good health and longevity, so, in randomised controlled trials, this can mean having to convince thousands of people to change what they eat for 20 or even 30 years. 'It's almost impossible,' Tim says. 'Humans change their diets all the time … So what we end up with is needing to look at lower-quality evidence to get an idea of how food can affect our health.'

Take one of the most expensive human studies ever conducted. In the early 1990s, the US government embarked on the Women's Health Initiative, which cost $625 million and recruited 160,000 post-menopausal women. One of the key components of the project was a dietary intervention, designed to test the ever-growing hypothesis that low-fat diets could reduce the risk of breast cancer, heart disease, and other serious illnesses.

Researchers enrolled 49,000 women aged 50–79, and put nearly 20,000 of them on a low-fat diet. But, in a follow-up after eight years of the trial, it became apparent that most of the participants in the low-fat group had been unable to stick to the diet they'd been prescribed. They were meant to have cut their fat intake from about 38 per cent of calories to 20 per cent. What really happened was they had only modestly lowered their intake, to an average of 29 per cent, which was insufficient to record any findings that could be deemed conclusive. 'The WHI, hence, failed to test its original hypothesis,' researchers from Harvard University wrote in 2015, 'and its null findings were largely uninformative.' The debate about dietary fat continues to this day.

In fact, decades of government diet guidelines recommendations on fat consumption (to limit total fat to 30 per cent, and saturated fat to 10 per cent) have very recently been called into question altogether. Why? In part, because it turns out that the longstanding hypothesis linking fat to heart disease overlooked randomised controlled trial evidence, and instead was drawn from a selective set of 'lower-quality' evidence that Tim talks about: evidence that comes from 'observational trials'.

These are the most commonly used studies in the field of nutrition. What observational trials do is track large groups of people over long periods of time, documenting what foods they are eating and the diseases that afflict them, and then attempting to determine any links that can be drawn between the two. These sorts of studies are not without scientific value. Easier and more practical to run than randomised controlled trials, they have proved useful in helping first reach some of the more unambiguous maxims we know today, such as *Don't smoke*, *Go easy on the booze*, and *Keep a healthy body weight*.

Observational studies work when it comes to larger effects. The risk of lung cancer for long-term cigarette smokers, for example, was established in observational studies as being 20 times greater than for non-smokers. But when it comes to hypotheses about more nuanced potential risk factors in nutrition — such as the very specific effects of the consumption of lots of red meat, or chocolate, or fish oil — there is a massive problem. Unlike randomised controlled trials, observational trials are not controlled experiments. There is no *intervention*. Participants are not made to alter their diets at the outset of the trial. Scientists can observe that people on different diets have different health outcomes, but what about other things that might be at play? For instance, what about the participants' socio-economic class, the type of work they do, or their exercise habits? Is it possible to isolate a specific element of their dietary intake from all of the other potential influences? This is where they are problematic. Observational studies, at best, can only help demonstrate association, not causation. They cannot prove a clear, causal link.

(Randomised controlled trials into the dangers of tobacco would be impossible, because scientists cannot intervene and force people to take up smoking. But for many years, and despite overwhelming observational-study evidence all coming to the same conclusions about smoking and lung cancer and heart disease, this limitation allowed Big Tobacco to dispute the consensus by arguing that statistical links don't constitute proof.)

Being healthy is, of course, a very common aspiration. And everyone eats food. So it is little surprise that news coverage of the latest nutritional research ranks especially high in the public interest. The headlines are everywhere: *Stroke and dementia risk linked to artificial sweeteners; Eating fried potatoes doubles risk of death; Mediterranean diet may slow the ageing process by five years; Coffee cuts risk of dying from stroke and heart disease.* Look a little closer, though, and many of these mainstream-media nutrition stories are coming from observational trials, which throw up all sorts of interesting associations, but are prone to being over-dramatised by journalists and bloggers alike. They are also prone to being contradicted by another study down the line. What this means is most of the nutrition research that consumers read is beset by major limitations. Some experts go so far as to say, 'If you find that [a] study was not randomised, we'd suggest that you stop reading it and go on to the next article.' With a scarcity of definitive research to road-test nutritional claims and hypotheses, consumers are often left to guess what they should be reaching for in the supermarket aisles. And, as the advice clashes with itself from one day to the next, a new phenomenon has emerged amid the confusion.

Under the banner of 'wellness', amateur nutritional advice readily available online has slowly seeped into the mainstream. Wellness, fuelled by the surging uptake of social media, Tim says, has transformed nutrition from a scientific discipline into a field where anyone can be considered an expert, as long as they have a good story to tell.

Well, not just *anyone*.

For the most part, this new breed of wellness gurus is white and female, young and attractive, engaging, and media-savvy. Some are yoga teachers, or personal trainers, or martial-arts instructors, but scant few have any qualifications that equip them to give health advice. What they do have is an Instagram account.

For the most successful wellness figures — those who have turned their blogging into a full-time job — a powerful story is a must. And the formula is always the same: zero to hero. It begins at their lowest of lows, and ends with enlightenment (and, of course, a desire to share the message they have learnt). The story is often their biggest selling point. Their blogs and websites all lead with it: perhaps they got sick; maybe a loved one had a brush with death. Bloggers with a point of difference — they might claim to be self-taught, or be curing their illness, or travelling the world taking inspiration from local cuisine, or snapping their own cookbook-ready photos — are the ones who really make it.

From their varying social-media pages, these wellness gurus document their lives online, posting an endless stream of highly curated shots of themselves, and of food, and of themselves with food, and of themselves just generally living well. Their food looks perfect, and so do their lives. What they claim to show is a transformation: weakness to recovery to empowerment. They aspire to inspire health of body and mind, self-love, boosted confidence, the best version of yourself. They can now amass thousands, sometimes millions, of fans. Along the way, they earn book deals and product endorsements. They might not say it outright (though some do), but with most of these bloggers the inference is very clear: a byproduct of all of this wellness is weight loss. But striving for wellness is far more attractive than *dieting*.

In an online world where food fads and conflicting theories abound, 'wellness' bloggers purport to light the path. The advice they're peddling is not all bad. Wellness bloggers promote a focus on healthy, fresh food. You won't hear them encouraging cheeseburgers, French fries, or sugary soft drinks. But these are people whose credentials are often measured by nothing more than their own personal experience and the number of followers they have collected. They are pseudo-experts, reliant on pop-science and opinion and a disregard for facts. With a ready-made platform operated out of the palm of their hands, they often dish out advice that is not only wrong — sometimes, it's plain dangerous. The sick and the vulnerable are ripe for exploitation. The rise of the wellness blogger embodies one of the most worrying cultural trends of our time: the unstoppable spread of misinformation on the internet.

Belle Gibson wrote about the detoxification properties of the humble lemon and how that made her think about the importance of diet. 'I decided then that if all I had was between one hour and a month to live,' she said, 'I was not going to spend it passed out on the hospital lawn, knee-deep in nausea and other side effects. I pulled myself out of chemo and radiotherapy — my doctors freaked out, but they couldn't stop me.' She also listed the non-negotiables in her diet — fluoride-free water and food that was vegetarian, as well as gluten, dairy, preservative- and refined-sugar-free — the foodstuffs she categorised as the 'start of all crankiness and illness'.

Gibson's statements on the internet were more extraordinary. She posted on Instagram in December 2013 that Gubinge, a type of Australian plum found in the bush that's high in vitamin C, was a superfood 'capable of healing cancer'. In a post about noni berries, she wrote that some studies suggested the fruit could 'reduce cancer cell reproduction, slowing down tumor growth, with the possibility of reversing and assisting in cancer treatment'. In response to a credulous fan who reported feeling bloated, Gibson said 'cutting out gluten, sugar and dairy is a must'. She diagnosed another person over Instagram as being dehydrated or having a mineral deficiency, and prescribed Himalayan or Celtic sea salt. 'And maybe bake some sliced sweet potato with some of the salt sprinkled on top,' she told her. 'Table salt is bad but mineral rich salts are incredibly good for you.'

Gibson gave advice about skin conditions and Irritable Bowel Syndrome in which she recommended 'probiotics, kombucha and sauerkraut … along with cutting dairy, wheat and sugar out entirely'. And she dumbed down nutrition advice. In one post of her holding a pink smoothie, she said the drink would target a rash caused by her liver cancer, inflammation caused by flying, and help boost her immunity and brain function. In one of her more blunt posts about treating terminal cancer, she wrote: 'I gave up on conventional treatment when it was making my cancer more aggressive and started treating myself naturally. I have countless times helped others do the same, along with leading them down natural therapy for everything from fertility, depression, bone damage and other types of cancer.'

This is a Western-worldwide phenomenon. In the US, one of the most well-known wellness bloggers is the Food Babe (real name,

Vani Hari). Hari, who was once a management consultant, has no training in nutritional or food science, and yet has risen to the ranks of being named by *TIME* magazine as one of the most influential people on the internet (her website records millions of hits every month). She has a book about dumping toxic food and living a healthy lifestyle, a *New York Times* bestseller in 2015. Her journey to nutrition began after a poor diet landed her in hospital, she says, and, like the other bloggers, she taught herself everything she knows. She's now a prominent activist who campaigns against Big Food companies — taking on the likes of Subway and Starbucks — and declares her life's mission to be raising awareness about 'what's really in our food, how it can affect our health, and how a handful of large corporations are poisoning us for profit'. Experts widely accuse her of being alarmist and misrepresenting food facts to suit her agenda. One described her as 'utterly full of shit,' and said her writing was the 'worst assault on science on the internet'.

In England, twenty-something Ella Woodward started blogging around the same time as Belle Gibson. Five years later, the wellness blogger had more than 1 million Instagram followers. The daughter of politician Shaun Woodward and Camilla Sainsbury (of the supermarket-owning family), Woodward, too, says it was illness that spurred her on to learn about a healthy diet and lifestyle. The poster girl for healthy eating is self-taught, although it was reported in 2016 that she was training to become a nutritionist. Woodward now runs a small food empire — a series of bestselling *Deliciously Ella* books (her first earned the title of fastest-selling debut cookbook of all time), an app, two London delis, and stock on shelves in major department stores. And it's all grown out of a bunch of recipes that are vegetarian, wheat-free, and refined-sugar-free.

But Woodward, once described in *The Guardian* as the 'author of arguably the most successful fad diet cookbook series in recent years', has been criticised for being part of the 'clean-eating' fad, which experts say can fuel an unhealthy relationship with food. Other British wellness personalities to be lumped into this category include the glamorous Jasmine and Melissa Hemsley — aka the Hemsley Sisters. The self-described 'home cooks', who also aren't trained to give health advice, built their business off the back of a service 'helping people with their digestion and relationship with food, and teaching the importance of gut health'. Their books were international hits, and they now have a TV series on Channel 4 in the UK, and a café at Selfridges on Oxford Street in london.

To top it off, there are the fashion models and the movie stars. Gwyneth Paltrow, on her website, goop.com, has promoted everything from a week-long goat-milk cleanse to vaginal steam cleaning. She's recently tapped into the lucrative supplementary medicine space, launching Goop Wellness, a line of vitamin supplements for women with catchy names like WHY AM I SO EFFING TIRED? (costing $90 a month). It's one of the latest additions to Goop's virtual shopping aisles, where health-conscious customers can trawl online galleries for products promising to help achieve better skin, stronger nails, shinier hair, and cleaner insides. Among them is a green powder said to contain 39 superfoods, beauty dust to 'glow from within', and something that allegedly supports you 'in accomplishing physical or entrepreneurial feats'.

Paltrow has written about detoxes and juice fasts and elimination diets, and has released the inevitable line of cookbooks. Her second book, based on a diet she adopted after her own health problems led her to the realisation she was intolerant to certain foods, contained only recipes that were free of dairy, eggs, sugar, meat, soy, coffee, alcohol, and deep-water fish. Reviewers slammed the book for promoting quack science, and The Guardian described it as 'food-phobic'. But, while Paltrow's health advice consistently raises eyebrows among experts, she is leading the charge of Hollywood celebrities making inroads into the wellness movement.

On the corner of Fifth Avenue and East 28 Street in New York City, two blocks from Madison Square Park, there is a training academy inside a 26-storey edifice. Some of the best-known faces of the wellness world have completed its courses to become what the academy calls a 'health coach'. However, most recent graduates have never set foot in the midtown office block. The year-long course offered by the Institute for Integrative Nutrition is now run solely online. Among its most high-profile Australian alumni are celebrity chef and paleo-diet crusader Pete Evans, former magazine journalist and *I Quit Sugar* author Sarah Wilson, and the late 'Wellness Warrior', blogger Jess Ainscough. Model Miranda Kerr has also said she studied there, being schooled in the academy's philosophy of adopting a holistic approach to food, relationships, exercise, career, and spirituality.

According to its website, IIN teaches graduates about 100 different dietary theories on top of coaching and business development. But questions have been raised about its online structure and the quality of its curriculum. Critics say the course has no foundation in the teachings of anatomy, physiology, nutrition sciences, and biomechanics — put simply, how the body works. They say graduates are in no way equipped to give nutrition advice, and point to the years of full-time study that dietitians, by comparison, have to undertake before they are able to assess, test, diagnose, and treat patients. Sarah Wilson, for one, is upfront about this. On her website, on a page dedicated to promoting the academy (where she discloses that she earns a commission for every new referral), Wilson says: 'A health coach is to a nutritionist what a life coach is to a psychologist.'

But that hasn't stopped Wilson, who advocates a no-sugar diet, from giving out what appears to be nutrition advice. In March 2017, her team responded to questions about her fruit-pyramid infographic that ranks bananas, watermelons, and dates among fructose-high options that should only be eaten 'sparingly'. After criticisms of the pyramid, which experts roundly described as 'stupid', 'confusing', and 'without basis', Wilson's website published a post clarifying the point: quitting sugar was just 'a gentle experiment' with yourself. 'While we offer guidance, we don't do strict rules — because even though we ALL need to limit added sugar, we're also all different!' it said.

Pete Evans, who lives by the paleo diet (which, against health authorities' dietary guidelines, bans dairy, grains, and legumes), has also written cookbooks with a hefty serve of nutrition advice, without having any real expertise apart from his personal experience. Described by his own television network as 'Australia's most controversial chef', Evans has also drawn criticism for his alternative views and for giving medical advice online. One of his books, *Bubba Yum Yum: the paleo way for new mums, babies and toddlers*, was dropped by publisher Pan Macmillan in 2015 after health authorities launched an all-out war against the TV chef over a homemade infant-formula recipe containing livers and bone broth, which they warned could potentially kill babies. Evans subsequently self-published the baby paleo cookbook with a revised version of the recipe. It carries a disclaimer warning that relying on the contents inside could cause 'negative health consequences'.

Evans, who has more than 1.5 million likes on his Facebook page, has said that the paleo diet can help shrink tumours and lead to cancer remissions. He claims the caveman diet can also help with medical conditions, including autism, asthma, and Alzheimer's disease. The late Gerson Therapy advocate Jess Ainscough, who sold more than 10,000 copies of her book, also came under fire for promoting quack science. Ainscough — who, unlike Belle Gibson, actually had cancer — might have believed she was healing herself from the terminal disease with nutrition and the controversial therapy, but the truth is, she wasn't.

Around 10 years ago, T. Colin Campbell, a Jacob Gould Schurman professor emeritus in nutritional sciences at Cornell University in Ithaca, New York, gave a guest lecture to students at the Institute for Integrative Nutrition. The video-recorded lecture — delivered before it became an online-only school — was uploaded to its website and kept there for some years. Then, one day, Campbell asked for it to be taken down. The academy obliged.

In 2012, Campbell released a statement denouncing the school. He had delivered the speech at the request of an old student, he wrote, but said he left with the feeling it was a dangerous, yet profitable, operation. He believes it should not receive any professional recognition in the teaching of diet, nutrition, and health:

> The speaker roster included a mixture of professionals and non-professionals, some of whom had serious conflicts of interests and some of whom pretended to be authorities when they were not. There is no question that there is a great need for public nutrition information but I strongly believe that this program does more harm than good. The fact that the students are led to believe that they are credentialed in this subject is a disgrace. I am very much sensitive to the public's participation and interest in this topic but enrolling in this lecture series is, in my opinion, a huge waste of time and money.

The year-long course at the Institute for Integrative Nutrition costs US$5,995. If you send the academy an online inquiry about tuition, the admissions staff promptly initiate the hard sell, sending daily email reminders urging you to sign up to secure your limited-time-only seat and take the first step to 'improving the world's health and happiness!' They offer a payment plan at 15.99 per cent interest, and also list external finance options, including credit cards or personal loans through banks and credit unions. 'Some people ask a loved one to sponsor them through it and then pay them back interest free or split monthly payments with them until they start seeing clients,' prospective students are told.

Increasingly, dietitians are reporting having to spend their time correcting misinformation that clients have been fed by wellness bloggers. The Dietitians Association of Australia has set up a page on its website titled, 'Challenging Misinformation', regularly posting responses to inaccurate and misleading stories in the press. But the message still isn't getting through. The association's Clare Collins says this is because of the plethora of conflicting advice available online, because changing eating habits is hard, and because people are drawn to a quick fix.

'If someone says you only have to do this magic thing, that is very appealing,' says Clare. 'Just don't eat sugar, or just eat like a caveman, or just eat all natural foods, and your cancer will be cured.'

Take, for instance, one of the most vilified ingredients on the market today: gluten. Sales of gluten-free products have soared in recent years, but between 1 and 2 per cent of the population actually has coeliac disease, a serious medical condition that causes all sorts of gastrointestinal problems. Certainly, many people have varying degrees of gluten intolerances that might not necessarily amount to being coeliac, but research also shows that consumers are cutting out wheat, rye, barley, and oats from their diets after self-diagnosing intolerances that might not even exist.

The advice from experts is the same: focusing on one single food villain is a dietary concept that is deeply flawed. And that doesn't just apply to dumping ingredients such as gluten or fructose or lactose. It cuts both ways. Before introducing certain foods, consumers should think carefully about what they're been fed. Because, increasingly, it's a marketing buzzword that's being used to drive up the price of products said to contain extra nutritional benefits. Food isn't just food any more. It's *plant-based food*. It's *whole food*. It's *superfood*. The bombardment of blog entries and attention-grabbing media articles promoting food myths make it all the more difficult to decipher fact from fiction. We're inundated with listicles (articles that are simply lists of things) promoting the benefits of walnuts and salmon. But are these foods *really* any better for you than other types of nuts or fish? Is pink Himalayan sea salt a healthier alternative to regular salt? Is quinoa any more nutritious than plain old kidney beans or lentils?

'If there's a fruit or vegetable that's spruiked as being picked by nymphs before the sun rises on some special hills, then be highly suspicious,' warns Clare, 'because you can already hear the cash register going *ka-ching, ka-ching*.'

The best nutrition bodies around the world invariably have the same core message: drink water; keep saturated fats, added sugars, and alcohol to a minimum; eat fruit, vegetables, whole grains, dairy, lean meat, and fish (or a suitable vegetarian alternative). Yes, lots of processed food is bad for you, and yes, fresh juice — pressed or blended — is good for you. But the difference between a handful of spinach and a handful of kale is negligible. Eating a punnet of berries — whether they're blue or red, or have a marketing plan based on a myth — won't make a bit of difference. And the entire concept of a detox diet or a cleanse to help achieve long-term health is plain nonsense. (The liver and kidneys already perform this function, and the best way to help filter toxins is to not overload the body with processed foods and excess kilojoules in the first place.)

Since the late 1990s, there has been a term given to the condition afflicting people with an unhealthy obsession with healthy eating: *orthorexia nervosa*. And hospitals are treating more and more people who are depleted in important nutrients because their diets are too restrictive. Researchers are now studying the phenomenon, believed to be driven in large part by fad diets, the obsession with presenting the best version of ourselves on social media, and a willingness to dump entire food groups without even the slightest scientific explanation. One nutritionist believes the fearmongering food advice served up by unqualified bloggers is driving such eating disorders. In a popular post on her website, titled *The Superfood Wankery List — Top 5*, Tara Leong, from the Sunshine Coast in Australia, tries to debunk the nutritional myths around some foods. Açai, she says, contains about the same amount of antioxidants as an apple. Coconut, technically a fat, will not help with weight loss. And rice-malt syrup is a sugar with the same amount of calories as normal sugar. She ends the post on a positive note. Topping her list of *real superfoods*, she writes, are 'basically any fruit' and 'basically any vegetable'.

— 8 —

PINK BALLOONS

Oli's fourth birthday party was late on a Sunday afternoon, and sunlight streamed in through the large windows of Gibson's Elwood home. Gibson had organised gold foil balloons in the shape of the letters 'O' and 'B'. Lego and other toys were strewn across the floor, and presents and handwritten cards piled up in the dining room next to party bags. Outside, on the patio table, were healthy snacks and a cask of filtered Pureau Water.

There were about a dozen kids and some of Gibson's closest friends at the party. Nathan, Oli's dad, was there, as was Clive, her partner, who wore dark sunglasses inside. Also present were her photographer, her food stylist, and a young woman named Kate Bradley, an author, who would go on to become Gibson's assistant. Jarrod Briffa and Bec Villanti, who ran a city café, and Georgie Castle, the founder of vegan chocolate company Citizen Cacao, had come along, too. A five-year-old boy with brain cancer, Joshua Schwarz, whom Gibson had met through social media, was there with his father.

For all of the criticisms that have been levelled against Gibson, everyone who has known her agreed that she is a devoted and loving mother. The former friend who lived with Gibson in St Kilda when Oli was a toddler said she was a 'terrific parent' and 'born to be a mum'. 'She always put him first, always wanted the best for him,' the woman said. Clive, too, has been described as a doting and attentive stepfather. 'He has a really beautiful relationship with Oli,' said another friend. 'Really gentle and caring.'

The party started out as a nice day, guests said, and Oli was having fun playing and running around with his friends from kinder. Nathan helped light the candles on his son's green Lego block before everyone sang Happy Birthday. Just before the speeches, in the dining room, Gibson had Oli on her hip, and looked at her son adoringly. Oli is a lot like his mum; he has the same fair skin and sun-streaked hair. He wore a long-sleeved T-shirt with a dinosaur print; she wore a $1,000 dress under a pink turtleneck sweater. Later, Oli knelt on a chair at the head of the table and excitedly unwrapped his pile of presents as his friends looked on.

Just after 3.15 pm, as people prepared to leave, Gibson's eyes rolled back into her head. Her legs buckled and she hit the wall, sliding down it, slowly, to soften the impact. As she lay on the ground, Gibson started shaking. At first, no one knew what was happening. Then she started convulsing. 'It was scary,' said one of her friends. 'It was so violent, the adults were crying.'

One guest pulled out her mobile phone, primed to call an ambulance. Then the seizure stopped. Someone said Gibson didn't like getting hospitals involved. 'It was, "No, no, no, this has happened before, everything's going to be all right, she'll get through it,"' said another friend. 'There's no need for an ambulance. That was the consensus.' Gibson came to, and explained to her guests, wearily, that this happened all the time. They shouldn't worry. But then the fitting started again. It went on for 30 or 40 minutes: Gibson seizing on the floor, and then coming out of it. When she stopped jerking, she seemed almost unconscious. 'People were stroking her forehead, reassuring her, "It's OK now, it's over." And then it would start again.'

Oli and some of the other children had seen the beginnings of the seizure, and the adults crouching around Gibson, cradling her head. Then someone took the little ones away. 'Oli was … I saw his face,' said a friend. 'He was petrified. The kids had to almost walk over the top of her to go upstairs. Oli had to look at his mum looking like she was almost dead on the floor.'

One of the guests, someone who was very close to Gibson at the time, said what they had witnessed left them absolutely devastated: 'It looked real. I believed it was real. And I was mortified. I cried driving all the way home … I actually don't know how I got home.'

Later, at home, Gibson updated her status on her personal Facebook account, telling everyone of the dramatic end to Oli's party. And, as always, she used the opportunity to encourage others to share. 'I collapsed in pain and had multiple seizures over the following 40 minutes,' she said:

> This is the worst I've ever been with them and am taking this overwhelming situation as encouragement to breathe and sort some things out. For anyone who's been in a situation like this before, I would love to hear your management strategies, whilst I send you love and strength in return. I have seizures often as a result of my brain cancer, but nothing ever this long or intense. Extremely grateful for my friends and family who were there to support me through this and my team who are looking for new answers.

***

On 29 July 2014, a little over two weeks later, Belle Gibson uploaded her most prolific post to Instagram. It featured a photo of a bouquet of bright pink balloons, in the shape of a love heart, captioned with the heartbreaking announcement that her cancer had spread to multiple organs:

> With frustration and ache in my heart // my beautiful, gamechanging community, it hurts me to find space tonight to let you all know with love and strength that I've been diagnosed with a third and forth [sic] cancer. One is secondary and the other is primary. I have cancer in my blood, spleen, brain, uterus, and liver. I am hurting. As some of you remember, there was a scare I briefly spoke about here 4 months ago where we found gynecological cancer that I stood up against with strength I wouldn't of had if it weren't for each of you. With these, it was only a matter of time before it all fell apart as my body goes through the waves of this process. I wanted to respectfully let you each know, and hand some of the energy over to the greater community, my team and TWP — through this I am still here reading, listening and learning with and to each of you, but need to respectfully and with great honour hand it over to TWP to carry on our legacies and collective message. I sit and work from a space for each of you, still creating and growing our philosophy of living #thewholelife — work towards releasing our first book and ensure that the legacies of our charity and community work which you ALL helped achieve through downloading The Whole Pantry App is all it needs to be, with whatever ends up being my defining story with you. I'm doing okay, but am feeling very unwell and picked up on this before my return from NYC with confirmation just over a week later. I have the most phenomenal team of integrative and holistic specialist and practitioners and know either way, they'll give me good conversations to leave with. I'm so grateful for them,

my strength over the last five years and for being what seems to feel like the most unfortunate, tested life ever. Please turn to this account, the app and book in this time of space for our message of The Whole Life, app and book updates and community support and inspiration to continue on.

Please don't carry my pain. I've got this. x Belle

There was an enormous outpouring of grief. Tens of thousands of people read the post. Thousands upon thousands more commented:

You are such an inspiration and although you've got this know that there are so many here supporting you, too. Sending so much love and healing energy and thank you for [all] you have done, you are such an inspiration.

Kick that cancer's butt sweetheart!! You've done it before and can do it again!

Sending you lots of love and light @healing_belle. I know you are receiving the best treatment. I will be thinking of you.

Our thoughts are with you beautiful lady — you are an amazing soul and an inspiration to all around you. Sending all our healing energy your way xx.

All my love @healing_belle it breaks my heart to read this news. You have changed so many lives with your courage and strength and I pray you will beat this once again. You're an inspiration precious girl, take care and rest up.

'In my prayers sweet @healing_belle,' wrote self-help author and life coach Tara Bliss, a close friend of Jess Ainscough's. 'Please everyone, spare a prayer for this light beam.'

Sydney mother Lisa Kelly wrote that she was inspired by Gibson to start her website, Kids Health Australia, which curates information from both conventional and alternative medical experts. 'Wishing her and her little boy all the love and hope in the world,' she posted.

In Apple and Penguin's offices, the grave post was being brought to the attention of the staff working with Gibson. The head of Lantern, Julie Gibbs, emailed her team of eight the next day, copying in Penguin's then chief executive, Gabrielle Coyne. 'Last night,' she began, 'Belle Gibson posted this photo on Instagram and with it she told her community that her cancer has returned.' Julie said Gibson was determined to front the disease head on and that she was being supported and cared for. 'Our book remains incredibly important to her and she is even talking about the next one,' she said:

> Chantelle will be working with Belle to make sure the message of the book campaign is about how this incredibly healthy lifestyle has prolonged Belle's life — way beyond what was ever predicted by her doctors. We have an exciting social media and print led campaign and we know a huge number of her followers are waiting for this book. As ever, Belle will continue to communicate how she is travelling on her cancer journey. Belle is now ensuring that her movement, The Whole Pantry, has its own impetus and infrastructure that will continue her amazing work around the globe. She will continue to be closely involved as she can.

Gibson was perched on a stool at the long, communal table. She was dressed in pants and a top, and had on a pair of high-heeled sandals. Her guest, a well-known artist from Bondi Beach, had flown into Melbourne for work, but had made time to catch up with Gibson over lunch to talk about the possibility of collaborating on a new project. They had never met in person; they'd just started talking on Instagram a few months before. The meeting was two days after Gibson's announcement on Instagram that her cancer had metastasised, spreading from her brain and penetrating her blood, liver, uterus, and spleen. It was at 1.00 pm on a Thursday at Brothl, a Hardware Street café set up by Joost Bakker, the Melbourne entrepreneur whom the *New York Times* has dubbed the 'poster boy for zero-waste living'. Bakker's kitchen made stock for its soups from bones that were leftovers from some of the city's best restaurants and destined for the bin. The café was a favourite of Gibson's. She ordered for herself and her guest: broth, served in a glazed terracotta pot, chickpea falafels with sour cream, and flavoured kombucha. The pair talked business over lunch in the middle of the busy city laneway eatery.

Gibson, by now, knew how to leverage her following. Sales could always be better and she had come up with a way to inspire people to get excited about shopping for arrowroot, dulse flakes, adzuki beans, and all the other rare ingredients in her recipes. She wanted the Sydney artist to create beautiful labels that customers could print out and stick on to jars in their pantry. The idea was to make the process of planning and shopping for the meals more attractive. At first, the ingredient labels would be free with any app purchase, and then, later, customers who already had the app would be able to go online and buy them separately. Gibson told the artist that all profits would go to building wells and hospitals in Africa. The artist would work for free, designing almost 100 labels, but in return Gibson promised to promote her through The Whole Pantry's social-media accounts. Gibson had something everyone wanted: a league of followers, the backing of Apple, a book deal with Penguin. The artist knew that aligning herself with this social-media darling was a smart business move. 'This was before influencers and before people were buying followers on Instagram,' she said. 'It would have been great exposure, and exposure was everything.'

Over lunch, Gibson opened up about her health, her latest 'diagnosis'. At one point, the artist recalls, Gibson broke out in what she thought was hives. Then, as a woman seated nearby rose to leave, she passed Gibson a folded serviette with a handwritten message written on it. 'Thank you for being an inspiration to me,' it read. 'Shine on xxx.'

According to the artist, Belle started crying.

During their meeting, Gibson spoke 'expertly' to the artist about holistic treatment, and gave her advice about natural remedies and foods she claimed cured certain medical conditions. On her recommendation, the artist visited Gibson's acupuncturist in Melbourne the next day. The pair talked about the artist's father, who had just been diagnosed with bowel cancer. She said Gibson gave her advice for her dad, but never suggested he stop conventional treatment. Gibson told her it was important that he keep seeing his GP, but to get second opinions and be open to other treatment options. 'I didn't expect that,' the artist said.

Gibson also spoke about suffering from seizures, how it was part of her condition. 'She said usually they would only last five or 10 minutes, but one time she had a 40-minute seizure and developed psychic abilities afterwards. That now she could feel people's auras, and figure out what was wrong with them in a health sense. She said she saw a friend recently who she knew was dying, but she wasn't going to tell them because they were going to die anyway and she couldn't stop it.'

Something about her meeting with Gibson didn't *feel* right to the artist. 'But I felt so guilty for even thinking it.' She flew back to Sydney and got back to work on growing her business. In the end, she heeded that feeling. She never did the work for Gibson, and stopped replying to her emails. 'She's a very, very clever girl,' was her assessment. 'She's very convincing, almost too clever for her own good.'

It was around this time that doubts about Gibson's cancer story started circulating. Questions were being asked on the internet. People started posting comments about Gibson's story: how it seemed to lack important detail; how her lifestyle didn't seem to reflect the deteriorating health she reported online; how she managed to outlive her doctor's prognosis for a type of cancer that is so, so aggressive; how she didn't follow any cancer organisations, and never called for more funding to support brain cancer research:

This lady Belle Gibson, Instagram 'famous,' says she has terminal cancer and is healing/has healed it with eating raw food and lemon juice detox or something like that. Is this lady for real? I mean, obviously not, but really. Her whole story stinks and she never gives any detail about her health issues.

In what loopy motherfreakin' universe, I wonder, can a recent manifestation of secondary cancer ... be defined as a journey to wellness?

I have brain cancer and it generally doesn't spread to other parts of the body because of the blood brain barrier. My father had blood cancer and it makes you very ill and your immune system very low and yet somehow Belle is jetsetting around the world

and swimming in dirty pools in Bali. Further, she doesn't seem
to be having any treatment for any of the other cancers she's been
diagnosed with. I have been observing Belle and I have noticed a
lot of inconsistencies in her stories. I am not convinced Belle is
telling the truth about her health.

I did find it very strange that after making that one post about
the horrible deterioration of her condition, there is not one other
mention about her health anytime after that. Directly after, there's
a 'thank you for your well-wishes' post, and then it's vegan donuts,
salt scrubs, crystals and twee. Something doesn't add up.

Yeah, don't forget sponsored cruises to Nouméa as well, just 3
weeks ago. This smells.

Has anyone heard of Belle Gibson at all? I am 99 per cent convinced
she is a fraud. I have brain cancer which is why Belle's story first
caught my attention. Brain cancer is aggressive and incurable and
it CANNOT be left untreated for 5 years. It is a rare disease and at
this stage very little is known about it—it most certainly cannot
be cured/treated by eating super-foods, practicing meditation etc.
I wish it could be, believe me! Belle is a businesswoman NOT a
cancer patient. Belle Gibson is a fraud and she is fooling the world
and winning awards and it is truly depressing.

One blogger began a post about Gibson like this: 'Does Belle
Gibson actually have cancer? Woah. Okay. Boy did I feel like a jerk
as I typed that out.'

But it was a question that some people who were close to Gibson
had already begun asking themselves. One young woman who had
become quick friends with Gibson was a very successful entrepreneur

based in Melbourne. She planned to go into business with Gibson, launching a range of superfoods. In March 2014, they got as far as registering the business with the corporate regulator. Both women were listed as directors. But the more time the woman spent with Gibson, the more ill at ease she felt about the person with whom she was considering a professional partnership. She remembers sitting in her accountant's office with Gibson, and both being asked to produce some basic paperwork. 'And Belle said, "Oh, that might be an issue",' she recalled. 'And the accountant was like, why? And Belle said, "Because I have several names that I go under". Then she said she was in witness protection, that it was a long story. At another point, the accountant asked, "What's your overall goal for the company," and Belle answered, "World domination."'

The woman also found it odd that she was finding out personal information about Gibson through social media. This was someone she considered a good friend, so she was surprised to get updates about her health on Instagram before being told about it by Gibson face-to-face. And there was another side to her friend. She said Gibson would present an all-natural personal online, and then do things like eat at McDonalds and drink alcohol and take diet pills. Once, when they were in an elevator together, Gibson complained that 'the pressure hurts my tumour'. Finally, there was the pink balloons post: 'I found that a lot of things that she had said just didn't quite add up, but that was just unbelievable,' she said. 'I got in so much trouble with my friends for saying stuff like that I didn't believe her.' The woman distanced herself from Gibson, and then cut all contact. Their business never made it past the planning phase.

While holidaying in Bali, Gibson logged onto Facebook. She seemed defensive. She tried to explain that her health crises were as severe as ever, even though she appeared to be so well. She described, in detail, in case anyone doubted her, how sick she was: 'I have cancer,' she said in a status update:

I have damage to my major organs. I have an infection in my spinal fluid. I have swelling behind my right eye making it painful to see or open it. I have seizures; sometimes three times a day, sometimes three times a week. I have extreme issues with my reproductive system because of losing a child at five fucking months pregnant. I have been really unsupported this whole entire time and now that I have my fucking hair back, aren't poisoning myself with chemo, have a job and do 'alive people things' I'm suddenly okay and my limited support is entitled to disregard my emotions, needs and situation even more? Total bullshit. If you don't want to acknowledge it, don't. If you do want to acknowledge it, then be present; don't give me some not even second rate but tenth rate bullshit fluff support just for the sake of appeasing your own guilt, curiosity or conscience. I'm sick and heartbroken and if you aren't comfortable with this; please go away — right now. I'm okay and out of hospital here in Bali. Even a private doctor with some side background in German medicine was overwhelmed by my situation. People need to get real. It's so important to be selfish and to love yourself, find time for happiness and things that make you thrive — but also important to be selfless and think about and give to others. If you haven't got this balance, disappear and take time to love yourself so you know how to give love to others. This is relative and the voice of so many people with a chronic illness. Please keep them in mind, too. We need love, not comparison or toxic personalities.

Many of the people we spoke to for this book said that even if they did have a niggling feeling about Gibson, a feeling that her story didn't quite add up, they never thought she was lying about having cancer. Those who knew her described Gibson as having little quirks. They noticed little facial tics or a far-away look in her eyes. Half-a-dozen people reported seeing her break out in a blotchy hive-like rash. When she spoke, and when she wrote, Gibson often muddled her words. She could be vague, easily frazzled, forgetful. At the time, the friends believed these to be symptoms related to her illness. They just wrote them off. They thought she might have embellished the details of her upbringing. Maybe she was trying a bit too hard to elicit sympathy. But fake cancer? No. No one thought she would do that. 'There was a lot of things,' said one former friend. 'She would divert her gaze or she would stare right through you. Everyone just thought it was brain cancer. When you look back it's like, *Oh, that's not cancer, that's lying.* But even if you thought she wasn't telling the truth, who is going to be the person who turns around and says, "Hey, that 25-year-old single mother with brain cancer is lying."?'

One person involved with Gibson around this time was her first assistant. She worked for the young mother in early 2014, helping out on the app and planning the book. She was never particularly close with Gibson, but they were friendly enough and got along. 'I just believed that she was someone who was really ill, someone who was an inspiration, and I just wanted to get on board and help her,' she said.

It did not, however, take long for her to realise that Gibson didn't really understand what she was talking about. According to the former assistant, when they were researching content for the book, she would ask Gibson questions about the medicinal properties of certain ingredients, and would receive responses that were always very general. She said most of the time Gibson searched online for the answer, and took information about certain foods from Google and Pinterest.

The assistant was also privy to Gibson's schedule, and was surprised she did not seem to be receiving any medical treatment. 'She'd never go to the doctor, she'd never talk about her illness,' she said. 'She'd do things like post on social media that she'd been at the doctor's all day, but really she wasn't. I was working with her one day, and she got her veneers done, but she said she was at [the] doctor's for an appointment, making it sound like it was for a cancer-related illness.'

Later in 2014, Gibson took on another part-time assistant, Melbourne author and vegan cook Kate Bradley. Kate would become one of Gibson's closest friends, and would back her until the very end. Kate is from bayside Black Rock, south-east of Melbourne. She's in her mid-20s, and has long, dark, wavy hair. Like Gibson, Kate built her brand online. Kate gave up refined sugar, gluten, and processed foods in 2012, and started a website about healthy food. She earned a strong following on Instagram, and secured a publishing deal. Her book, *Kenko Kitchen* (Kenko being the Japanese word for health), was released around the same time as Gibson's. Gibson trusted Kate: she was the only other signatory on Gibson's business account. In the back of her book, Gibson describes Kate as 'a friend I'll have forever'.

The feeling was mutual. Kate was one of Gibson's most ardent supporters. Like just about everyone who had grown close to Gibson, she believed in her. But no one was more publicly invested. Kate was cited in one media article as one of Gibson's closest allies. And she could not have spoken more highly of her. 'Belle mothers like she has no other commitments or worries,' she said. 'She is here to change our lives and community and help people who have no voice or think they have no choice. She fights her battles every single day for the pure reason that she isn't done showing the world goodness.'

More than a year before Gibson was exposed, Kate posted on her website her top 10 health food inspirations. She named 'Healing

Belle' No. 1:

This girl is slowly starting to become a household name and for very good reasons,' Kate gushed. 'She is a warrior. She is a fighter. She is a survivor. She is a charity worker. She is very talented in the kitchen. She is extremely smart. She is a beautiful mother. She is a beautiful friend and she is just simply an awesome inspiring human being. I wish I was joking when I said this girl probably cares more about your health than you do yourself. She will not back down until she changes the world in every way that she can. This girl is a powerhouse who is determined to impact the health of everyone and the wellbeing of families and people across the globe. Her iPhone/iPad/Android application The Whole Pantry has changed the lives of many. Not for just the recipes, resources and articles making people healthier and giving them the confidence in themselves to change their lifestyles. But also for where the money goes afterwards. This girl doesn't pocket the money to give herself luxuries but instead puts it towards charities targeted at helping families of those affected with cancer, helping girls return to school in Sierra Leone, helping restore human rights to those forced to seek asylum and helping women give birth safely in areas where this would not before be possible. And the rest goes towards her next project, all aimed at impacting people around the world. This girl also has brain cancer, and has been battling with it for years. She was told she did not have very long at all to live at the age of 20, and whilst she started chemo and radiation she then flipped these treatments the bird and decided to do it her own way. Four years on and she has the medical world amazed by still standing strong, doing what she is doing with a tumour still sitting in her brain. Oh and did I mention she is just now 24? Belle is currently working on a book which I know will be revolutionary. Let's face [it], anything she does is. I can't give this girl enough props as she is just amazing. Anyone yet to download her application I recommend you do so. It is beautiful, filled with amazing things and very, very cheap. People just don't get better than her.

The week the news broke, Kate finally left Gibson. She distanced herself from the scandal, and deleted the glowing post from her website. She has never spoken publicly about their relationship, and has declined repeated requests for comment. Friends say Kate was devastated by Gibson's betrayal. 'She was really upset about the whole thing,' said one. 'She just felt like she'd being completely conned.'

—9—

THE INTERVENTION

Spring had arrived in Melbourne. The days were starting to lose their chill, but the evenings were still stubbornly cold. The weatherman was talking about temperatures as low as six degrees on the night that two of Belle Gibson's closest friends decided they were going to confront her. After dinner, around 9.00 pm, Chanelle picked up Jarrod in a Volkswagen SUV. They drove down Glen Huntly Road towards Gibson's townhouse, and all along the way they debated what to say once they got there. Could there be an explanation for Gibson's strange behaviour? And her muddied health claims that simply weren't adding up? Maybe. But rumours were getting around. People were turning suspicious. These two friends knew Gibson better than most, and, by now, they were almost certain she was faking. 'We've got to get her to come clean,' Chanelle told Jarrod. Gibson didn't know they were on their way over, so when they were five minutes from her house, they sent her a text message. They turned off the main road and into her tree-lined side street.

Gibson was a supreme networker. People, it seems, have always been drawn to her. She had a special eye for those with social clout or business nous, and an enchanting way of building strong relationships quickly. When Gibson went to parties, she brought her new friends along, introduced them to the host, invited them into her world. Some have described her as the kind of friend who made you feel good about yourself; the sort of person who inspired you, and pushed you to do better. She endeared herself to people; drip-feeding them secrets, confiding in them, sometimes crying with them, letting them into her inner sanctum. She was good at making people feel important. 'She was so secretive about her personal life,' said one person, 'so if you were allowed in, you felt really privileged.' With a couple of former friends, she'd got matching tattoos. But then there was another side. An unforgiving side. Even her closest friendships were often intense and almost always short-lived.

By this time, in 2014, Gibson had known Chanelle and Jarrod for a little over a year. Jarrod was in his late 20s, and was the co-founder of a popular city café called Kinfolk, a social enterprise staffed by volunteers and asylum-seekers, which gave its profits to charity. Pictures of Jarrod — bald, olive-skinned, with just enough facial hair to look scruffy yet sharp — had been featured in newspapers and on current-affairs shows, and he was becoming well known about town. Chanelle was about the same age as Gibson. She'd only just moved to the city, but the pair had become fast friends. A former banking analyst turned entrepreneur, Chanelle was petite and blonde-haired; sharp-witted and exceptionally strong-willed. But tonight, as she parked the SUV in Gibson's dimly lit street, Chanelle had knots in her stomach. Her heart was pounding, but she didn't waver. She wasn't the sort of person to sit by and do nothing when something didn't feel right.

Chanelle and Jarrod rang the intercom and waited. Gibson appeared at the door and said hello. She shaped her lips into a smile, but didn't look thrilled to see them. The door closed behind them, and they followed her in, along the wooden-floored corridor and into the large living area beyond. Chanelle and Jarrod sat on the couch beside the gas fireplace; Gibson sat down, too, and Jarrod looked her in the eyes. He let some seconds pass before he spoke. And when he spoke, his tone was serious. Was there anything Gibson wanted to tell them, he asked. Was there anything she had been untruthful about? Jarrod stressed that they were her friends and that they would support her. He promised they wouldn't judge her. But they needed to *hear the truth*.

Gibson looked confused. 'What?' she replied. She demanded to know what they were talking about.

'Are you sick?' Chanelle interjected, and, all of a sudden, there was no going back. The words that no one had dared utter before poured out of her mouth. 'Do you have cancer?'

Gibson's face dropped. 'Of course!' she demurred.

Chanelle can still recall the exchange that night, word for word. She started by asking Gibson about the Instagram post — the one in which she announced that her cancer had spread to other vital organs. She asked her if she could tell them the name of the doctor who had given her the diagnosis.

'Dr Phil,' she said.

'Are you serious?' Chanelle was incredulous. 'Dr Phil?'

'He came to my house, and picked me up and took me to his practice.'

'Where was the practice?'

Gibson claimed she didn't know. 'He's now disappeared,' she said. 'His colleagues told me his practices were questionable.'

'Questionable?' said Chanelle. 'Doesn't that mean that your diagnosis is questionable?'

Gibson said she supposed it could be.

'Well, wouldn't the first thing you'd do be to go and find out what the *real* diagnosis is?'

'I don't have time.'

'What about for the sake of your son, to know his mother's not dying?' asked Chanelle, with upturned hands. 'Wouldn't you make it a priority to go to a hospital and find out the right results?'

Again, Gibson replied that she was too busy. She compared the situation to how celebrities should not have to confirm or deny gossip-magazine rumours about whether or not they were pregnant. She said she would go to the hospital for a diagnosis in her own time, when she was good and ready.

Chanelle left the room. She went upstairs and confronted Clive, Gibson's boyfriend, as he was coming out of a bedroom. 'I asked Clive to his face,' Chanelle recalls. 'I said, "Clive, you need to tell me the truth about Belle."'

Clive Rothwell, the curious partner of Belle Gibson, is described by those who met him as a private man: quiet, withdrawn, sometimes a little bit awkward. 'Very smart and very polite,' one person remarked. At parties and social outings, Clive was often in the background, never splashy or loud, never one to attract much notice. He's older than Gibson, about 40. He has short hair, and auburn whiskers that have started to turn grey. When they got together, Gibson was already claiming to have terminal cancer. Clive never prodded her about it; it was a sensitive subject, and he didn't want to stick his nose in. Even if he was puzzled about some inconsistencies here or there, they weren't enough to lead him to think she was not sick. What did he know about cancer anyway?

In the middle of 2014, that changed. Clive's father, Geoff, was diagnosed with cancer, and had only months to live. Clive and

Gibson split up for a while, and Clive packed up and moved back to suburban Adelaide to live with his parents. It was then, while Clive was *really* living alongside someone with the insidious disease, that he became suspicious of Gibson's story. Terminal cancer is merciless. Grotesque. It wasn't something that permitted you to thrive; at least, not the way Gibson had, all throughout their time together. Geoff Rothwell's funeral was held in the first week of September, in a small chapel, 15 minutes from his house.

It wasn't long before Clive was back in Melbourne, back with Gibson and back to being a stepfather to Oli. Several people who knew the couple well during this time have confirmed that Clive began openly questioning Gibson's diagnosis. 'He didn't say in so many words, "She doesn't have cancer",' a friend said, 'but he referred to it as a *fucking joke.*' Some former friends said Clive had tried to go to medical appointments with Gibson, but she would never let him accompany her. 'He would have to beg her,' one said. 'Then one time she let him, he dropped her off and drove around the corner and waited … and then he saw her cross the road to a park. She didn't even go into the hospital.' Others said that Clive believed Gibson was suffering from a mental illness, and that he tried to get her help.

'It was his dad's dying wish for them not to be together,' one said. 'I don't know why he's still there; maybe he still loves her. Maybe he's trying to protect the son.'

So here they were. Clive and Chanelle, standing at the top of the staircase, speaking in lowered voices. Gibson and Jarrod were still downstairs in the living room.

'*Clive … tell me the truth.*'

'He said, "I need to protect that little boy",' recounts Chanelle.

'I said, "Protect him from what?" He said, "She's not sick … and she will try to destroy anyone that exposes her."'

Clive pulled on a jumper and agreed to come downstairs to join the others.

Gibson, meanwhile, had called another one of her friends, a natural therapist, whom she had just started seeing. She wanted him to back up her side of the story. He lived on the other side of the town. 'You've got to come over,' she urged him. Half an hour later, he was at the front door. She made one more phone call — to her publisher, Julie Gibbs, in Sydney. Gibson seemed paranoid. She was beginning to think that Julie didn't believe her story anymore, and had been talking to her friends. 'What have you been saying?' she asked her over the telephone, in front of everyone.

'It was a panic response,' one person described it, but Julie reassured her that 'everything's cool'.

The five of them sat for some time longer, around the small coffee table in the lounge of Gibson's home. Jarrod and Chanelle were on the three-seater, Gibson in the armchair, the natural therapist on the armrest, and Clive on the floor. It was October, and Gibson's cookbook, *The Whole Pantry*, was weeks away from being launched in bookstores across the country. If her claims about her cancer diagnosis were wrong, or made up, it had to end now. Chanelle and Jarrod implored her to show them a *single piece* of medical evidence: test results, an oncology report, a brain scan, a scribbled note from a doctor, anything. Gibson replied that she didn't keep any of them. It was too negative to have that stuff around the house, she said. It made her too upset.

'I told her, "The book is about to come out, and people are going to pay money for that",' said Chanelle. 'People who are sick are going to read that. Do you really feel comfortable that that's going out to the world when you don't even know if your diagnosis is correct?'

At one point, Gibson turned to her natural therapist, imploring him to tell the others. '*You* know that I'm sick. *Tell them*!' The natural therapist was confused. He wasn't a doctor. He had always thought Gibson had cancer, but that was only because she had told him so, and he had no reason to think otherwise. He felt uncomfortable, and didn't know what to say.

Gibson sulked, but Channelle did not relent. She accused Gibson of lying, and the conversation started getting heated. 'This is your inner circle knocking at your door,' Chanelle said, her tone sharpening. 'This is where it begins, this is where it can end.'

'The other two were leading the questioning,' recalled the natural therapist, 'but I definitely thought something was off. She was avoiding every question; she said she didn't have any of the test results — she said she had left them with the doctor.'

By the time it was over, he doubted everything Gibson had ever told him, and ran through in his mind all of the peculiar stories she had told him in the past that hadn't sat quite right. 'She once claimed she had heart surgery,' he recalls, 'but then, when she wore a low-cut top, there was no scar to be seen. "Where's the scar?" I asked her.' Gibson had replied coolly: 'It was microscopic surgery.'

The guests left Gibson's house amicably. No one hugged or kissed her goodbye, though, like they usually did. It was close to midnight, and had become even colder outside. Chanelle and Jarrod got into the car, and they looked at each other, muted, dumbfounded at the gravity of what they had heard. '*Holy fucking shit!*' was all Chanelle could say. Their parting words to Gibson had been that they hoped she would decide to do the right thing. They had tried their best to stress to Gibson the importance of coming forward about her health doubts now, *before* her book's release. She was already in way too deep. But if she let the book come out, that would be it. You can't get rid of a book the way you can scrub history from the internet. Her lies would be enshrined in print, and there could be no turning back. But Gibson didn't listen to them. She said she felt unfairly victimised. She dug her heels in.

On the eve of the book launch, Gibson told Julie Gibbs that a jealous friend had turned on her. Internal files from the publishing house that would later be used in court make it clear that Julie understood this to mean there were allegations that 'Gibson had fabricated part or all of her illness.' But the book launch went ahead anyway. And on Thursday 23 October 2014, the false story was ordained by the world's biggest publisher.

The book launch was in a basement event space in central Melbourne, on Bourke Street, called Donkey Wheelhouse. The basement was beneath a stunning, 125-year-old Venetian gothic building that was once the head office for Melbourne's horse-drawn carriages and cable trams. The room was wide and high, and usually rents out for up to $1,300 an evening. Gibson's launch party was an exclusive affair. Ritzy and intimate. There were perhaps 80 people, and the bar was serving kombucha tea, colourful juices, and sparkling mocktails. Chanelle was among the guests, despite all that she knew. Gibson was standoffish with her for most of the night. Clive avoided all eye contact.

Gibson had gone for the '60s look; a cropped, monochrome top, skirt, red lipstick, and her hair styled in a puffed bouffant. Beaming attendees posted on Facebook their selfies with Gibson from the night. 'Some people are just amazing,' one wrote. 'That's Belle Gibson, and so humble, too. Can't wait to get into this book: not just a recipe book, but a total guide to healthy, holistic living … congratulations beautiful Belle.'

One of the very first to arrive at the party was Amanda Steidle. She was washing her hands in the venue's bathroom when Gibson, whom she had met once before, snuck up behind her and pulled her in for a hug. 'She said she was quite nervous,' Amanda recalls, 'a mix of nervous and excited.' Amanda, the founder of a 'Healthy Mums' weight-management program, was the first to have her new book signed by the star author, and they stood chatting for a while. Within minutes, it seemed, the crowd swelled and the party became considerably busier. Soon, guests were having to wait their turn for their moment with Gibson, or to ask her to autograph the book's front cover. Gibson drifted about the room, guests recall, 'a hello here and a kiss on the cheek there'. She whisked some of them away to the side to join her in the photo-shoot area. 'There was an air of excitement,' one said. 'Everything was buzzing.'

The buzz had been building for months, and the much-anticipated launch party did not disappoint. Guests were thrilled to be there, to be in the presence of the remarkable Belle Gibson. And, by all accounts, the book was a hit. There was, after all, a lot to like: from the emotional power of her story, to the simplicity of the recipes, to the elegance of the photography. 'It was beautifully put together,' said Amanda. 'I was impressed with how young she was and what she was doing, and I wanted to support her and the promotion of better eating.'

Among the better-known guests at the launch was 'dude-food' chef Dan Churchill, a former MasterChef contestant from Sydney's northern beaches: 'If you ever quit or feel like you should give up on something, I want you to think of this amazing young woman. So proud to be at your first book launch @healingbelle. The fact you say I inspire you is an amazing sentiment.' He posted the message on Facebook with a photo of him and Gibson posing together. Singer-songwriter Clare Bowditch, who couldn't be there, posted a message: 'Thinking of Belle launching her Whole Pantry book tonight, and sending good vibes! Smash it!'

Social media lit up that night, and in the days that followed, with gushing comments about Gibson and *The Whole Pantry*, accompanied by uploaded photographs of the book laid flat on wooden tables or on fresh-linen bedsheets:

> So excited we finally purchased a copy of The Whole Pantry cookbook by Belle Gibson. If you are unfamiliar with this inspiring young lady, please check out her incredible app. It's a great place to start if you are looking to make some changes.

> Congratulations @healing_belle and @thewholepantry team on the launch of this beautiful book. It was so lovely to celebrate this amazing achievement with you at such a heartfelt event. I am very excited to try some recipes, especially the buckwheat pasta. Big love to you all!

> Yup so got this in the mail today! #wholesome #thewholepantry. Can't wait to try. HealingBelle, thank you so much for being an inspiration in times of need.

Sarah Wilson, author of *I Quit Sugar*, posted a photo of a purple amethyst stone sitting on top of *The Whole Pantry*: 'This arrived in the post,' she wrote on social media. 'Healing_Belle you are a gem. Thank you for the big fat purple healing rock!'

The early reader reviews of *The Whole Pantry* were fast to follow. And all across Facebook and Instagram, there was not a single negative post to be found. People far and wide breathlessly shared her recipes on their pages: homemade sauerkraut, paleo bread, broccoli pesto, raw cacao, raspberry and beetroot muffins, roast vegetable stacks with cashew cheese.

Gibson's book was a unanimous hit, and the newly published

author was showered with adulation:

> I will be putting into practice some of her wonderful life practices
> to increase my health and well being.

> If you haven't heard of The Whole Pantry, Belle is literally a hero.
> She has no ego, and her motivation in the 'health and wellbeing'
> industry is heartfelt. An incredible human being who has to be the
> definition of courage, I am sure of it.

> I love the new HealingBelle #TheWholePantry cookbook so much
> I bought in bulk! Look away now if you're on my Christmas list.
> Ha ha! The love almost jumps off the pages.

> HealingBelle, you have outdone yourself! This is so much more
> than a cook book.

Midway through the launch party, publisher Julie Gibbs took the floor and cleared her throat. She made a speech about Gibson's courage; how honoured she was to work with her, and how inspired she was by her personally. Gibson followed, giving an emotional address. She started by thanking Clive and Oli, as she always did, and then she thanked Julie, and her food stylist and her photographer. She also thanked her assistant, Kate Bradley. She didn't thank Jarrod or Chanelle. Gibson's teary speech was about her journey with cancer and how happy she was to have made it through. 'She was lying the whole bloody time, and we were sucked in,' one attendee later said. 'I'm sickened by it.'

Leading up to the launch, Penguin's publicity arm had been hard at work. A sophisticated social-media strategy was developed. Media gift packs were sent out. A list of 'key influencers' was compiled — famous female models, authors, journalists, TV stars, singers, athletes. The book was to be featured across the Apple, Google, and Kobo websites. It would be a feature title in the Target catalogue, and Collins' and Dymocks' Christmas catalogues. *Vogue*, *Cosmopolitan*, *Marie Claire*, *Elle*, *Women's Health*, *New Idea*, *Sunday Style*, *Body+Soul*, and the *Design Files* would be offered stories. ABC Radio wanted an interview. So did the morning TV shows, and Channel Ten news. The plan was to launch the book in Australia, then the UK and US, and then it would be shopped around to other foreign publishers keen to translate it.

One week after the book launch, Penguin's external PR firm, Sefiani Communications, provided a draft 'contingency communications' document, a crisis PR plan, in case Gibson was ever accused of making up the story that had propelled her to stardom.

10

THE REAL-LIFE BELLE GIBSON

It's not hard to see the allure of someone like Belle Gibson: the hope she was offering people with cancer, and how good she looked doing it.

'It's confronting to most, even those attached to my life each day, that I get up and get on with everything,' Gibson once wrote on Instagram. 'That I "don't *look* sick".'

Meet Monique Watt, the real-life incarnation of what Gibson purported to be. In her mid-20s, a single mum, she grew up in Brisbane, lives in Melbourne, and is living with terminal brain cancer.

Monique once looked quite similar to Gibson. Sitting at her dining-room table in her home on the outskirts of the city, she picks up her iPhone and scrolls through the gallery of selfies: red lips and a button nose, toned skin, and sun-streaked hair. The last photo is one of her and her daughter, Siennah, in the family car. It was taken a couple of days before the cancer was found, on 20 July 2016. Monique doesn't take photos of herself anymore. She hates the way she looks.

'I can't stand it' she says, fiddling with her silver bracelet, 'I don't recognise who I am.'

Less than a year after she was diagnosed, Monique *is* unrecognisable. She has put on 30 kilograms, and none of her old clothes fit. She has a moonface, her neck and arms are puffy, and the hair on her head is thin and patchy. She is constantly battling the side effects of aggressive cancer treatment. She can no longer work, and survives on welfare. Monique set up a GoFundMe page to raise money for expensive immunotherapy treatment, which isn't publicly funded for people with grade-three brain cancer. At the time of writing this book, after the page had been live for more than a year, less than $600 had been donated.

Monique has just moved into a new rental house, one with no stairs, after a fall at her old place. This one is on the edge of the city, on the edge of a residential estate, just down the road from her mum. Her children aren't home, but there are signs of them everywhere: a wooden play kitchen pushed against the wall, and a high chair and fresh crumbs on the floor beneath it. It's an overcast and humid day, but every now and then Yarra Ranges sunlight slants through the blinds. Monique is wearing a purple-and-red Aztec-print top under a lightweight black shawl. She takes a sip from a can of Coke — the only thing that helps settle her nausea — and tells the story of the day she found out she was sick.

It was a Monday. Monique went to the doctor complaining of persistent headaches. She was prescribed pain killers, but by Wednesday she was vomiting from the sharp pain in her head. She couldn't hold the tablets down. Monique went back to her GP, and, right away, she was sent for a CT scan at La Trobe University Medical Centre in Bundoora. She was anxious — not about the procedure, but because Siennah wasn't allowed to go in with her; she had to sit in the waiting room by herself. After the scan, a nurse came in and asked Monique if she was feeling OK.

'Yeah, I'm fine. Why?'

'I'm just asking,' the nurse said. 'We're going to go do a contrast now.'

Monique didn't know it then, but the iodine-based dye being injected into a vein in her arm is what's used to get clearer pictures of tumour growth in cancer patients. Monique was scanned a second time. She was told she couldn't leave — the radiographer needed to speak with her. The reception staff had Siennah behind the counter, distracting her with pictures of different-shaped body parts on blue-and-black printed scans. That's when Monique suspected something was wrong.

'Have a seat,' the radiographer told her.

'What's the matter?,' she asked.

'We've found something on the scans. We believe it to be a large glioma. We're not sure if it's cancerous, but it could be.'

Monique's stomach lurched to her throat. Her mind went into overdrive. And she can barely remember what happened next. On the scan of Monique's brain, the cancer is easy to make out. It's lighter in colour than the rest of the tissue, a whitish-coloured mass with well-defined edges, shaped like a lunar crescent. Nestled in the front, on the right, it looks much too big for the space.

The rest of the afternoon was foggy. Phone calls to her mum and sister. Arranging daycare pick up for her two-year-old son, Elijah. Getting to the hospital after being told she wasn't allowed to drive herself. Being strong for Siennah, seven, who was with her the whole time. 'Within two hours of the scan,' recalls Monique, 'I was in hospital being told I probably had a rare type of cancer and that I might have to have brain surgery that night.'

Place your finger halfway across your right eyebrow. Go straight up to your hairline. This is where Monique's scar begins, where surgeons carved open her head. It's red, raised and then dented, and goes back diagonally, towards her ear. Here, just under the skull, the tentacles of a 3.5-centimetre growth were burrowing into her brain, slowly killing her. The tangle of cancer that was dug out is called a grade-three astrocytoma. It struck in Monique's frontal lobe, the part of the brain responsible for motor function, memory, language, judgement, and impulse control.

When the cancer was found, Monique had just split up with her partner, and was working as a disability carer. She thought her migraines were caused by stress. Then she started vomiting bile. Looking back, there were earlier signs of trouble: the ghostly pain that struck the right side of her jaw, which she'd put down to a toothache; the numbness in her left arm she now knows was partial paralysis; the memory problems (she'd recently left an airport without collecting her bag at the carousel); and the trouble she'd had sleeping and waking in the early hours of the morning, with severe pain in her head — both common symptoms of brain cancer. All these symptoms got worse as the tumour grew, causing her brain to swell.

It turns out that Monique has inherited a genetic condition called Lynch Syndrome, which made her prone to a number of different cancers. Most commonly, these tumours are found in the bowel and uterus. Monique's case is believed to be one of only a handful where the condition has led to cancer of the brain. Monique's family said her great grandfather died from brain cancer, when he was 34 years old.

Monique's grandmother, Wilma, flew down to Melbourne from Brisbane after the diagnosis to stay with her granddaughter. A full-time volunteer at the Ronald McDonald House in South Brisbane, she put her life on hold to be with her. In Melbourne, her days are packed. She ferries great-grandchildren around when Monique can't drive, and she runs the household. She's understanding, in that way that only grandparents can be with their grandchildren.

'Some days after the chemo, I'm in bed until 2.00 pm,' says Monique, looking across the table to her Nan. 'Some days, I don't want to go anywhere.'

Wilma nods. 'You just have to go with it,' she says, returning a warm smile.

The chemotherapy tablets that Monique takes are called Temozolomide — four blue capsules, 100 milligrams each, every morning for five days at the end of the month. Then she suffers with the side effects until the next round of treatment a month later. Add them to the list. On top of the weight gain (caused by the medication to bring down swelling on her brain and a month-long stay in hospital), Monique feels sick and tired, and she breaks out in rashes. Thick hair is gone from her head, but has sprouted on her forearms where there wasn't any before. The left side of her body is weaker. She's always hot and clammy, even when the air conditioning is on, and even when the rest of her family is rugged up in blankets on the couch. She has lost her appetite and, when she does eat, she gets bad indigestion, anyway. Heartburn is constant. So is feeling queasy. If she doesn't have diarrhoea, she is constipated. Monique is regularly struck down by what feels like bad period pain, even though she hasn't had a period in months.

The thing about brain cancer is that it cannot be cured. Not ever. It can be fought. The standard treatment for the type of cancer that Monique has is surgery, radiotherapy, and then chemotherapy. It can be cut out, and zapped and poisoned, but even with aggressive treatment, it always comes back, and always becomes a grade-four tumour, the worst kind. The Australian Cancer Council has put the average survival rate for people with Monique's cancer at three years. Brain cancer, although rare, is a certain death sentence.

'I'm going to have it forever and, at some point, it is going to kill me,' says Monique, her voice trembling. 'I don't know when, but it will. You don't survive brain cancer the way you can survive other cancers.' She looks out the glass sliding-door off the dining room, past the trampoline and beyond the wooden fence, where excavators are busy backfilling land for rows of new houses. They're going back and forth in unison, beeping and rumbling. 'I've looked at alternative medicines, because that's what you do when you get told you are going to die from cancer. I don't know if any of it would do me any good, but if I have the chance to try something that will extend my life, then I'll do it.

'I haven't been able to find anyone diagnosed with a grade three who has survived more than 10 to 15 years.' Monique stops talking. She takes a deep breath. 'I've not been able to find anyone.'

'You know,' sighs Professor Terry Johns, as he loops around his busy research lab. 'I wish I could give you a good message.'

But when it comes to brain cancer, the simple answer is that he can't. And neither can anyone else whose career is devoted to the fight against it.

Every November, towards the middle of the month, Terry gets on a plane to the United States to attend an important meeting, run by the Society for Neuro Oncology. Since 2008, he's been to just about every one of them; to hear from experts from the best universities and hospitals around the world, and to learn about what sort of advancements have been made. The last one he went to was in the desert city of Scottsdale, Arizona, at the Fairmont Hotel, a sprawling 450-acre resort with five swimming pools and two golf courses. There was a session on epigenetics in brain cancer; talks on the latest tumour classifications; and a series of question-and-answer sessions, lectures, and long panel discussions. Pulitzer Prize-winning author Siddhartha Mukherjee, known for his bestseller, *The Emperor of All Maladies: a biography of cancer*, gave the keynote address, and, on the Saturday night, all the conference's attendees were taken by bus to a gala dinner at an exclusive private airport nearby. In all the years Terry has been going to the conference, though, one thing has remained exactly the same: there has been no improvement whatsoever in brain cancer survival times.

'Not one bit,' he says soberly. 'Not one month. Not anything.

'It's not like we haven't made enormous progress in understanding the disease, the mutations, the genetics of it, the cause of it … but we just haven't been able to convert that information into change for patients.'

It's Monday morning at the Hudson Institute of Medical Research in the Melbourne suburb of Clayton, and Terry appears from the elevator, wearing a sensible shirt, untucked, and his wavy hair brushed to one side. He raises the swipe card on his lanyard, holds it to the reader that opens a big glass door, and so begins another week. The other scientists in his team are younger than him — they are mostly graduate students, in their 20s and 30s. Terry, 53, appears to have just as much zeal as any of them. Today they are working on the development of special antibodies that carry a powerful toxin. Known as ABT-414, these antibodies act like heat-seeking missiles, capable of homing in on brain cancer cells and destroying them, while avoiding healthy tissue. It's also not as toxic as chemotherapy, so patients do not suffer the same debilitating side effects. But researchers like Terry don't talk in terms like 'today'. You'll hardly hear them say 'this week' or 'this month'. They measure their progress in years. And sometimes in decades. Terry did the first experiment on these very antibodies 19 years ago. And only now are they in what's called a phase-3 clinical trial, which is finally nearing the very end of the drug-testing process. The trial is extremely expensive. It involves 700 patients in the US, Europe, and Australia, and costs hundreds of millions of dollars.

The patients on this trial all have glioblastoma — the most common and most aggressive kind of malignant brain tumour. Some have had what's known as a 'complete response' to the intravenous treatment, which, when it comes to brain cancer, is very promising news. It means that their tumours had completely disappeared before returning, and therefore prolonged their survival times. 'Some lasted two or three years before it came back,' Terry says, 'but there are just not enough of those patients at this stage to say it's a slam dunk.' His big-pharma industry financier, AbbVie, believes the drug has a good chance of getting approval in 2018.

In the complex field of brain cancer research, experimental trials like this one are slowly emerging, which is a good thing, because the stakes could hardly be higher. Most people who get brain cancer will die very quickly. Doctors often rank different cancers by the likelihood that a patient will still be alive five years after they are diagnosed and start treatment. The reason for this is that five years is considered a sort of benchmark after which patients are considered to have a better chance of their cancer not returning. Around two-thirds of all cancer sufferers will make this milestone. But when you narrow in on brain cancer patients, less than one-quarter live five years. Most will be dead in a year or two. On the list of cancers with the worst survival rates, malignant brain tumours are very near the top.

'If you get colon cancer, surgeons can take two feet out of your colon, absolutely make sure you've got every bit of the cancer out,' Terry explains. 'You can chop out 70 per cent of the liver and still live. If you get it in your kidney, you can chop out one kidney, and you've still got the other.'

Chop out a chunk of your brain, though, and you could be left paralysed or severely impaired. One wrong incision can erase memory, language, motor skills. Cut out the wrong chunk, and you are dead. Brain cancers have a habit of infiltrating brain tissue with tiny finger-like tentacles of malignant cells, which become enmeshed in the brain and cannot be safely extracted. So when surgeons remove brain tumours, there are always small pockets of cells away from the main cells that get left behind. If a patient has 99 per cent of cancer cells removed, they can go into remission, 'but 1 per cent of a tumour of a trillion cells is still quite a few of them,' Terry says, 'and 12 months later it comes back more furiously than the original.'

In May 2015, at the Crown Palladium on Melbourne's Southbank, TV host Carrie Bickmore was named the winner of Australian television's top individual honour, the Gold Logie. She walked up to the stage to a roaring applause, looking glamorous, her platinum blonde hair draped over her shoulder.

'I know you all want to party,' she began, 'and you all want to go to bed if you're watching at home. But I'm going to use the two minutes that I have up here … to talk about something that's incredibly close to my heart. I want to talk about brain cancer.'

The 34-year-old stifled tears as she spoke about her late husband, Greg, who was killed by his brain tumour five years after being diagnosed. She put the golden statue down at her feet, and pulled a no-frills, bright-blue beanie over her hair.

'It kills more people under 40 (than any other cancer), and that's a lot of you in this room,' she said. 'It kills more kids than any other disease.'

Carrie Bickmore was correct. Brain cancer is *the* most expensive cancer. Not just for the individual, but for the community. With 60 being the average age of its victims (meaning roughly half of all sufferers are younger than that), it claims a higher proportion of healthy lives than does any other form of the disease. While survival rates for other cancers have improved dramatically in recent years, its prognosis has not budged since the 1980s, when radiation first started being commonly used to treat cancer.

Brain cancer strikes down people in their prime, forcing them out of employment, onto welfare, and causing a huge impact on their families. When it comes to children, brain cancer is second only to accidents as the leading cause of death. The outcomes for children's brain cancer are better than for adults, but treatment often leaves neurological defects. On top of the poor prognosis, brain cancer patients also face a lower quality of life while they fight to survive. This is partly because the cancer is attacking the most vital organ, and partly because of the devastating effects that treatment has on the brain.

If research dollars were allocated based on the burden of the disease, it is estimated that brain cancer would be in line for about twice as much money as it currently attracts. In the same year that authorities in Australia launched legal action against Belle Gibson, a federal Senate committee was set up to investigate funding for research into cancers with low survival rates, with a focus on brain cancer.

In the days after the Logies speech, Cure Brain Cancer Foundation's Barrie Littlefield attracted attention when he said brain cancer didn't get enough funding or awareness. 'It's not a "sexy" cancer,' he said at the time.

Two years later, he told us, 'There are no two ways about this: the system has failed people with brain cancer.' Barrie was born in the UK, and lives in Sydney. He used to work for big pharma, but, in 2011, his daughter, Eloise, 10, was diagnosed with a brain tumour and subsequently died. He is devoted to the fight against brain cancer, but says more funding is desperately needed.

'Watching your child die of this disease is not pretty,' Barrie says, bluntly. 'Kids, all their organs are new …' He pauses. 'And they hang on and they hang on, but they can be in great pain. My daughter, at one point, was screaming for me to kill her.'

'It's unacceptable for anybody to be dying of this now. We have the technology, we have the capability. We just need the focus and the funding. We know that with focus and funding, we can get survival rates up. Breast and prostate and other cancers prove that.'

The Cure Brain Cancer Foundation, founded by neurosurgeon Charlie Teo, has a mandate to lift the five-year survival rate to 50 per cent by 2023, and is currently funding about two dozen research projects around the world.

'There have been hundreds of trials in brain cancer that have been unsuccessful,' says the foundation's head of research strategy, Michelle Stewart. 'We are scouring the world for the best research projects that we think will have the highest probability of success.'

When Terry Johns was a student in his 20s, studying melanoma and multiple sclerosis, researchers shared stuffy lab spaces, and ran their experiments on their little allotted corners of the bench. Nowadays, the machines and microscopes in use are so specialised that you have to travel through an entire building during the course of a single morning. A tour of Terry's workplace covers three floors over a whole wing of a new state-of-the-art medical facility. And every year, he has to find at least $750,000 in grants just to keep his lab going. 'That takes a lot of my time,' he says candidly.

Terry takes the lift to Level 4, gets out his swipe card again, and opens the door to speak with one of his researchers, 35-year-old Sameer Greenall, a PhD who has been in his team for the past six years. He comes to work in jeans and a long-sleeved T-shirt. Down a microscope, brain cancer cells don't look nasty. Terry and Sam are growing some in small plastic dishes inside the lab. They were taken from a patient with a glioblastoma. Sam describes what he sees down the lens as a 'sheet of cells'. Up close, it looks like a thin layer of honeycomb.

In the next room, Sam hunches over a computer screen and opens an image file. What he's looking at now are scans showing the brain's own natural defence system — cells that line the walls of capillaries — which basically spit out drugs that are trying to get in. It's yet another reason that brain cancer is such a 'bastard'. 'Getting drugs into the brain has always been a big challenge,' Sam says. 'It's a very frustrating disease.'

But what's more frustrating, Sam explains, is being unable to offer any meaningful intervention while seeing how much patients suffer. Brain cancer is a different type of cancer. It attacks the 'essence of who you are … When you start to lose those faculties, and see yourself waste away. It must be terrible.'

In neuro oncology, Terry Johns is a well-known name. Sometimes, cancer patients will type his name into Google and phone him up at the office, asking what's the best trial to go on.

'Professor Johns, are you going to cure me?' one asked him recently.

Terry has to say 'no'. He tries to do it tactfully — 'We are working very hard, although you will not get cured' — but people often refuse to accept that there is no answer.

Terry and Sam say there is a unique desperation when it comes to cancer — to try absolutely everything. 'There is even more desperation with brain cancer,' Terry says. 'It's 18 months, often, from the minute you find out until you die. People do a lot of homework, spend a lot of money, and chase a lot of things down because they believe that if they do all the right things, they'll get cured. But the answer is, they won't.

'They will always believe they are the odd one out … And that's something Belle Gibson tapped into.'

Late on a hot night just before Christmas 2016, Monique's daughter, Siennah, crawled into bed with her. The seven-year-old wanted to know if her mother was going to die. 'She said, "Mum, you're not going to go to heaven, are you?" Then she added, "I want to go with you."' Monique's face turns red as her eyes well up. She folds a tissue in half, holds it across her eyes, and lowers her head into the palms of her hands. 'I didn't know what to say to her,' she says, sobbing softly.

Wilma is watching her granddaughter as she talks to strangers across her kitchen table about her own mortality. Her hands are clasped together on the table. 'From time to time, that still comes out,' Wilma says, 'where she'll say, "I'm going to live with my mummy all the time, I'm not going to get married."'

Monique manages a little laugh as she dabs her eyes with the tissue. 'Yeah, she says, "I'm never moving out of home. I can't leave you alone, Mum."'

The sound of earth-movers reversing travels through the window from over the back fence. Monique's priority is to spend time with her children, to make special memories with them. Knowing how to tell them about her illness has been her biggest challenge as a mother. 'What do I say to my kids?' I don't know what's going to happen, and I can't give them answers. Siennah thinks that if my hair grows back, everything is good, I'm better now, that's the end of everything. But she doesn't know.

'There's no end to this, except for certain death.'

11

THE TIP-OFF

'I spoke to the girl who was wanting to come forward,' the text message said. 'Her lawyers scared the crap out of her about slander. Check out healing belle on Instagram — or Annabelle Gibson — the girl who is cancer scamming.'

We heard rumours about Gibson in early 2015 through from a former colleague. Tips like this come into newsrooms all the time: allegations of a crime, a scandal, a complex cover-up. Often, the better they sound, the less likely they are to carry weight as a story. Like Chinese whispers, by the time a tip makes its way to a journalist, it has often morphed into something else entirely.

The young woman wanting to come forward was Chanelle. Before speaking with her, we expected an aggrieved former employee, or something like that. That's what they usually are. This would most likely amount to a non-story. The call to Chanelle was made between assignments, standing in line at a noisy café. Phoning her was more a matter of checking this tip off the list: hear her out, determine she most likely had an axe to grind without a shred of proof, leave it there, and then move on to the next story. After speaking with her, we felt very differently.

Chanelle lives in Sydney, but once lived not far from Jess Ainscough. She knew the 'Wellness Warrior' socially, as well as others in the wellness movement. Chanelle's dad is a detective, and her mum works for a cancer charity for women. Chanelle first met Gibson at The Whole Pantry launch in St Kilda, in December 2013, and was moved by her speech about overcoming cancer. Chanelle was writing for a magazine at the time. She wanted to interview the remarkable young developer for a story. Before long, they were friends.

Our first phone call went for well over an hour. Chanelle didn't seem angry, or to be acting out of malice. More than anything, she seemed afraid of what might happen if Gibson's business continued to flourish; if she was given even more of a platform. It was immediately obvious she was thinking about others. And she was very clear about what she wanted: 'To stop her.'

Going to a journalist with a story like this is a courageous decision; one that involves continuing commitment, hours upon hours of conversations. Chanelle had already approached another reporter with the story, but she had never heard back. So she got right to it. She told us about her doubts, about Gibson's seizure that she believed was fake, about the intervention, and about what Clive had said to her. Chanelle was sure Gibson did not have cancer. She believed she was a fraud.

Then she spoke about one of her mother's friends, a woman who had cancer and, after months of conventional treatment, had started looking into alternative therapies. Chanelle, at the time, could hardly have been more encouraging. She told the woman about her new friend in Melbourne, the incredible Belle Gibson; about how she had dumped chemo and radiation therapy, how she empowered herself, and how she had managed to stave off brain cancer with nutrition. Her mother's friend eventually made the decision to stop chemotherapy. A few months later, she was dead. Chanelle understands that there is more to this woman's death than a word of advice she'd offered, but she can't shake the feeling that she is partly to blame. Every time Chanelle talks about this, her demeanour changes. She becomes very quiet, and struggles to hold back tears.

We pulled everything there was on Belle Gibson: newspaper articles, magazines write-ups, blog entries, social-media posts, morning TV appearances. It was always the same. Gibson was a 'bona fide inspiration'. But it was immediately clear that the details of her life were always vague. There were no specifics: no family or friends quoted, no locations, no hospital names, no specialists. Nothing that we could cross-check. We bought her book at a shop not far from Gibson's house. The woman at the counter had to plug the title into her computer to jog her memory, but when she saw the cover on the shelf she recognised it immediately. 'Her story is amazing,' she said.

Back at *The Age* building, in February 2015, we took the book, and printouts of her articles and interviews, into a quiet room: the spring 2014 volume of *Peppermint* magazine, with Gibson on the front cover, and a two-page story, 'Food for Healing'; a glowing 1,700-word *Sunday Style* article, 'I Don't Feel Like I'm Dying,' which begins, 'Instagram is full of inspirational quotes, but few ring as true as those posted by @Healing_Belle.'; a clipping from the *Sydney Morning Herald*, 'Australian app developer's triumph,' which contained an extensive interview with Gibson, speaking at an Apple conference.

We scanned every sentence, examined every claim, every anecdote, one at a time. We pored over her public statements in previous interviews, speeches, and television appearances. Over the course of a few days, the misgivings we had about her story were difficult to contain. There were details that she kept repeating, about health, hospitals, cancer, and diagnoses. But they all seemed too scripted. They didn't *sound* natural. They didn't ring true. Her recollection of having a stroke at work seemed strange. The way she said her doctor broke the heavy news about cancer — 'You're dying … you have six weeks … four months' tops' — was especially difficult to swallow. And, besides, when it all came down to it, she simply had never looked like a sick person. She didn't look like someone with a death sentence hanging over her, with metastatic cancer coursing through her blood and her organs. She looked entirely the opposite: the very image of happiness, vitality, and bursting good health. No photoshopping required.

We found what we could from what was publicly available. We pulled her business records: *Belle Gibson* was the director of three companies, called Luxe Superfoods, Luxe Superfoods Group, and BG Luxe; *Annabelle Gibson* was the director of Belle Gibson Pty Ltd, and director and secretary of The Whole Life Pty Ltd. We ran searches on her associates, and we title-searched the houses she lived in. We scoured her social-media footprint to find whatever we could about her life before she came to Melbourne. There wasn't a whole lot; next to nothing, in fact, that could tie her to any job, or to any place, for years at a time. As we were doing all of this, her social-media posts started disappearing before our eyes. We learnt that she had just set her account to private.

If being vague and imprecise was Gibson's strategy to avoid any audit of her health claims, one of her best-known posts on Instagram from the previous year turned out to be her biggest misstep. A screenshot of the detailed Instagram announcement, from 29 July, the one announcing that her cancer had spread, was key. We compiled a summary of her cancer claims to date, added the latest details, and started sending it around to oncologists, to see if it checked out. Most wanted nothing to do with the story, but some, fed up by charlatans who sell false hope to their patients, said they would be happy to help. The first was a leading medical oncologist in Melbourne. He examined Gibson's claims. 'Sounds totally implausible,' he told us, but he would not go on the record: 'I'm very sceptical about the story.' A hospital brain surgeon, one of the best-known in the city, also agreed to examine Gibson's public statements about the nature of her cancer. He was unequivocal: 'It doesn't add up,' he said.

Before long, we had five people in her inner circle telling us they had doubts about her diagnosis. They all said the same thing: they'd never seen her sick; had never seen her with a doctor; had never seen her take medicine; and they believed she faked the seizure at her son's birthday party. We kept calling around. We spoke to people she knew, people who followed her around. Everyone thought it was possible she was faking, but nobody wanted to be the person to call her on it. If she didn't have cancer, they all said, it would come out eventually.

Everything was pointing to the one conclusion: Gibson's story was false. If we were writing about a more benign subject matter, we might have pulled the trigger. But these allegations could hardly have been more serious. This was a story about faking cancer and building a global business off the back of it. What if the people we were talking to were simply wrong? What if her disease was a one-in-a-million? What if, despite the way it appeared, she was just a young, innocent mother, who was dying from cancer?

We ran it up the chain, and then called *The Age*'s lawyers. Their answer came back quickly. No. Unless these people were willing to put their name to the story, they told us, it couldn't run. We agreed.

As much as we were convinced that Gibson was lying, journalists can't just access copies of people's medical records. The risk of getting it wrong was far too great.

But this didn't kill the story. We asked ourselves, *If she's lying about this, what else would she lie about?* Our chief-of-staff, Tom Arup, gave us a few days to dig around, a rare liberty in the understaffed and overworked 24/7 newsrooms of today. A starting point for our prodding was, in the end, a pretty obvious one: her claims of fundraising large amounts of money for charities.

We didn't have to look far. Gibson plugged her philanthropic work everywhere she went.

'A large part of *everything* the company earns is now donated to charities and organisations which support global health and wellbeing, protect the environment and provide education to those who otherwise wouldn't have the opportunity,' Gibson writes on the third page of her book. 'It's become fundamental now.'

In one glowing write-up, she was said to have given away at least $300,000 to various charitable causes all over the world. Everywhere we looked, Gibson said something different about her philanthropic pursuits. Sometimes she claimed to give away 25 per cent of her company's profits; other times, it was everything. In a bio she prepared so that Penguin could promote her book at the London Book Fair in March 2014, Gibson wrote that 95 per cent of her app proceeds went to charity. Nine months after her first fundraiser, from which she still hadn't passed on the money, Gibson lambasted other businesses for giving away just a fraction of their proceeds. 'In our worst month,' she boasted, 'where, I think we made $700 on the app, we still donated 25 per cent of that.'

On social-media postings in 2014, she wrote that a portion of *all sales* of the app would be donated to charity. The year before, she said 100 per cent of app sales for one week would be donated to the parents of a boy with terminal brain cancer.

On an Instagram post where Gibson responded to criticism about flying in first class, she claimed it was a 'free upgrade', and said she didn't keep any profits from The Whole Pantry. 'I don't actually use or keep any app money,' she wrote. In yet another post, Gibson wrote that she was 'working with over 20 charities'. In a first-person magazine article, Gibson claimed that the charitable side of her business which started off as an initiative to give a large portion of app sales to 'rotating charities' had since 'evolved to giving almost all profits' away. 'You have a choice to create a mini revolution in your life,' she wrote. 'We are working towards building two schools, have heavily invested in maternal health care and human rights ... and give donations and support to families in the TWP community whose children need holistic support throughout their cancer or medical treatments. Our love and hands are all over the globe.'

In a video interview at an Apple smartwatch event in California, she spoke in detail about the 'giving back end' of her company. 'Your app download transfers into community donation, so not only are you choosing to create changes within your life, you're also financing us to be able to support changes to those that otherwise don't have that access.' When Belle Gibson lies, she does it with a smile. She's charismatic, and looks her interviewer in the eye. She continued: 'So that's everything from funding medical support for children that are living with cancer to building schools in Sierra Leone.'

We tracked down people who had been on the invite list to her app launch and fundraising event, in December 2013, at the St Kilda White House. These were people who'd put cash in the glass bowl on the table; people who'd bought tickets online to the 'virtual' event. The invitation listed the charities Gibson supposedly supported: One Girl ('Help us rebuild a community school in Sierra Leone — when a girl is educated, everything changes'); the Birthing Kits Foundation ('Give women in developing communities a safe and sanitary space to birth'); the Asylum Seeker Resource Centre ('Restore human rights to those forced to seek asylum'); and the Schwarz family. ('Joshua, 5, has a terminal brain tumor which can't be operated on. His family are hoping to fly him to Mexico as a last resort for treatment.')

'We all have a lot of love and fire behind us,' Gibson told her guests, 'it'd be great to create some big beautiful change this weekend. Three dollars buys a birthing kit, $300 a school scholarship. No one needs to feel as though they can't take part. Accumulative effort has a massive impact.'

Then we found posts about online appeals, including a Mother's Day fundraiser. Gibson had pledged to donate proceeds from app sales to two charities working in south-east Asia. She praised her supporters for 'raising a further $5000' for the causes. 'Don't forget,' she said on social media during the campaign, 'for every app downloaded until this Sunday, your purchase goes straight to The 2h Project and the Bumi Sehat Foundation to prevent maternal and infant deaths. Tell me what family means to you … and I'll donate an extra $1 on your behalf. The potential is huge, but you have to get involved to change the world with me.'

We contacted all of the charities named by Gibson, one by one, and asked if they knew anything about her. Had they ever heard of her company, The Whole Pantry? Had they ever received a donation either from her or her company?

'No donation. Nothing,' said Kevin, from The 2h Project.

'We've had a look and we can't find anything under her name,' said Fiona, from Birthing Kits Foundation.

'I can say with confidence that we have never received a donation from Belle Gibson,' the Indonesia-based Bumi Sehat Foundation stated.

'Unfortunately, despite a number of requests to follow-up with The Whole Pantry to find out when we might receive the donation, we haven't received a timeframe for its transfer or the donation itself,' said Chantelle, from One Girl.

The Asylum Seeker Resource Centre, which had one entry of a $1,000 donation under Clive's name about a year earlier, said: 'Nothing further at our end. We're not really holding our breath for the money.'

Finally, we checked with authorities. Neither Gibson nor her company were lawfully registered as fundraisers. Consumer Affairs Victoria explained that people misrepresenting fundraising events could be in breach of criminal law.

This was a story we knew we could run.

It was a Thursday afternoon. First, we called Gibson's partner, Clive. When he answered, he was very calm and very cautious. We told him the reason for the call, and told him we would be contacting Gibson with a number of questions. We asked about his involvement in The Whole Pantry. Clive spoke slowly. He wanted to know what the angle of the story was. It was about Gibson's health and fundraising claims, we told him.

'OK. OK,' he said.

'I've being told by a few people that you've actually mentioned to some people that she wasn't sick.'

'Right,' Clive said.

'Is that true?'

'Well, not exactly, no,' he began. 'So, first of all, I don't really have anything to do with TWP, so in terms of any donations or anything like that, that would have to go through a business inquiry. In terms of Belle's health, uh, really she's the only one that would know any particular details about that.'

'You've been her partner for a few years, though, haven't you?'

'Yes.'

'And you live with her?'

'Yep.'

'OK. I don't mean to put you on the spot here … but the only reason I'm calling is because some people have said you told them she's not sick.'

'That's quite concerning to me, based on the fact that, um, really, somebody's health or somebody's condition is quite a personal thing, and, really, the fact that people would be speculating on that or putting that in kind of a public context is kind of an issue, I think.'

'And that's the purpose of calling you, to test the allegations. That's why I'm asking the question.'

'My take on everything that goes on is: Belle chooses to put certain things out into the public, which leads to scrutiny, leads to conjecture, and obviously people are going to ask questions. The way I see it is, anything health-related will be purely speculation unless it's a medical professional that can give their opinion, and I'm far from that.'

'But we both know, Clive, that you have an insight into whether she's gone to appointments, [had] reactions to certain treatments, or medical records.'

'Yeah, of course. So really my concern is Oli. He's Belle's son. That is my first and foremost concern. Obviously, Belle is also my concern. As far as the business or any of that kind of stuff goes, and any scrutiny that comes under, that will obviously come out in the wash in whatever way that it needs to.'

Clive then said Gibson was travelling interstate to attend a funeral. He politely ended the call.

We called Gibson from *The Age* newsroom, but her phone was off. She was on the way to the Sunshine Coast to attend Jess Ainscough's memorial service, which was being held the following day. We typed out a list of 21 questions:

Why have you not passed on the charitable donations you promised to the Asylum Seeker Resource Centre, the Birthing Kit Foundation, One Girl, the Schwarz family, The 2h Project, and the Bumi Sehat Foundation? If you have made donations to these organisations under any other name, can you please provide evidence of this by way of tax receipts or formal acknowledegment from the organisation? If the funds were never received by these organisations, then for what purpose were they used? In your book, you say 'a large part of everything' the company earns is donated to charities supporting health, education, and the environment. Which charities have received donations from TWP? For the record, can you also please clarify the following: What is your age? (You have said your age is 26, but your company records show that you have given your DOB as 8/10/91.) In your book, you said your cancer had been stable for two years, but months earlier you told media and posted on social media that it had spread. Can you please clarify which of these statements is false and what your current health condition is? At which facility in Perth were you diagnosed with cancer in June 2009? What was the name of the cancer you were diagnosed with? What stage was it? What was the precise prognosis? At which facility did you receive chemotherapy and radiotherapy treatment? What is the current status of your cancer? Will you provide the name of the doctors that you said in your book you see on an annual basis?

We mentioned our deadline — 2.00 pm the next day — and then hit 'Send'. The email was delivered at 3.20 pm on the Thursday. Gibson immediately hit the phones. At 3.30 pm, she called the Asylum Seeker Resource Centre in Footscray. She spoke to its director of fundraising for 15 minutes, apologised for the misunderstanding, and promised to pay them $20,000. At 4.01 pm, she transferred $1,000 to One Girl, the charity that had been chasing her for its promised donation for more than a year, and then sent a screenshot of the internet banking receipt from her phone to its CEO. She fired off emails to the other charities, too.

Then, at 1.16 am on Friday, the day of Ainscough's service, Gibson responded to our questions. Her reply was 1,500 words long.

'Thanks for reaching out,' it began.

We worked our way through the email. It failed to answer any of the questions properly. Gibson kept spruiking her charity work, wrote about her sacrifices for others, and her support for those less fortunate. This was odd. Usually, when people are caught out like this, and a reporter comes knocking, they say very little. Or they bunker down and say nothing at all. Gibson, on the other hand, attempted to explain away the fact that she kept money raised for charity. She said it had something to do with 'cash flow' problems. Even more bewildering, Gibson promoted the $1,000 donation to One Girl. She had transferred it to the not-for-profit less than 10 hours earlier, 15 months after she took it, and only after she was asked what happened to it.

Her email claimed the company was running at a loss, and that it had appointed external accountants, who had advised it to put a hold on all donations until their records were up to date. 'The financial priority is to still give this monetary support to those organisations we are invested in and care about,' Gibson said. 'To touch on your email, a previous employee was responsible for communicating with some of the charities you listed and it is unfortunately not to our surprise that this didn't happen.'

Gibson said the 2013 app launch only raised $730. Of the glass jar into which people put cash at the event, she said the takings only amounted to 'a few hundred dollars', which were passed onto a struggling family. She said money was given to other families, too, but did not provide any evidence of this. In reply to our queries about the Mother's Day Campaign, Gibson said $2,790 was raised, which, she felt was not enough to be split between the two charities she named. Therefore, she said, it had been *allocated* to the Bumi Sehat Foundation, an organisation that had never heard of her. Gibson further claimed that she planned to donate 'up to $20,000' to a birthing kits organisation, but provided no other details.

To the lingering question of the *large part of everything earned* that was donated to charity, she said: 'It was with nothing but good intention that we publicised the fact that a percentage of profit from the app will be donated to charity. With the benefit of hindsight, we now understand that there is a large difference in the perceived financial success of the app and the actual net proceeds received. Because of the slim margins and small amounts involved in app sales, donations will be subsidised by TWP book sales, the proceeds of which are due to be paid in October as per Penguin policy.'

By this stage, Gibson had earned almost half a million dollars from the app and book advance. We confirmed that Gibson did make *some* donations. They totalled just under $6,000. That included a $4,823 water-filtration system for her friend Jarrod Briffa's café, Kinfolk, and the hurried $1,000 donation to One Girl the day before.

We sent Gibson a second email, again asking the questions she hadn't answered: Where were you diagnosed? What was the prognosis? Where were you treated? We asked about the 'corporate' job she claimed to have, where she studied 'web development and business', and what her real age was.

In the morning, on her way to Ainscough's service, she wrote back.

'I am attending a funeral today of a close friend and someone who mentored me through many years, and so you will understand the brief nature of my responses,' she began. 'I have been very open and generous with the amount of personal information I have put out into the public domain and have been hurt by that. As such I am not willing to expand on that any further at this point.'

That evening, we emailed *The Age*'s lawyers, telling them we would steer clear of the health allegations and instead focus solely on the fundraising fraud. If we wre right — if the cancer was a lie — this article would smoke out the people we needed to prove it.

12

THE BACKLASH BEGINS

It was a bit after 8.00 pm on a Sunday night when the first critical news story ever written about Belle Gibson went live on the internet. The 750-word article was placed prominently on *The Age*'s website and, simultaneously, ran across all the news sites in the Fairfax Media publishing group: *The Sydney Morning Herald*, *The Canberra Times*, *The Brisbane Times*, and *WA Today*. We had been expecting the story to be held from the web until early the next morning, but one of the night editors in the newsroom that evening must have decided they needed some traffic:

'Inspirational' app developer's charity money missing
A social media entrepreneur who shot to fame off the back of her cancer survival story failed to hand over thousands of fundraising dollars promised to charities.

Melbourne businesswoman Belle Gibson, founder of food and health app The Whole Pantry, solicited donations from a loyal following of 200,000 people in the name of at least five charities that have no record of receiving money from her.

The 26-year-old's popular recipe app, which costs $3.79, has been downloaded 300,000 times and is being developed as one of the first apps for the soon-to-be-released Apple Watch. Her debut cook book *The Whole Pantry*, published by Penguin in Australia last year, will soon hit shelves in the United States and Britain ...

Ms Gibson has run two campaigns purporting to raise money for five charities, but Fairfax Media has confirmed that none has a record of receiving a donation. Four of the organisations, including Melbourne's Asylum Seeker Resource Centre, had no knowledge fundraising drives had taken place.

The Age, 8 March 2015

Like all journalists before a big story goes out, we were nervous. You go over every line in your head, making sure it's backed up. Defensible, if it comes to that. But we knew the story was solid. The charities had confirmed they never saw a cent from Gibson, and she had left a trail of fundraising promotions all over the internet. We weren't worried so much about Gibson. But we were bracing for the inevitable; an onslaught of abuse from her legion of followers, the kind of digital lynch-mob storm that has become so familiar in the social-media universe. To Gibson's community, she was more than a chic Instagram celebrity. She was an inspiration to them, and a hero. Many even spoke of feeling a spiritual connection with her. Her online presence was vast, and the fallout from this story was bound to be big. It was something we would much rather have dealt with once we were back in the newsroom in the morning. But that was out of our hands now.

It didn't take very long. Comments streamed in on *The Age*'s social media, and emails started trickling into our inboxes. Within minutes, an extremely long-winded rebuttal appeared on The Whole

Pantry's Facebook page, raising many of the dubious defences included in Gibson's responses to our questions. The central excuse seemed to be that the company's books were not up to date. It was written by Gibson, although she referred to herself in the third person:

THE WHOLE PANTRY — LIVE HEALTHY
8 March at 18:51

This evening *The Age* — theage.com.au posted an article which we have been communicating with them over the past couple of days. They contacted Belle, our previous Managing Director, who addressed some incorrect claims and assumptions but they still decided to run with the story without correcting factual errors. Unfortunately, the two journalists have been selective with their information, so here we are, updating you with where we are actually at.

We have, like all start ups, struggled with managing all facets of a new business, biting off more than we could chew, juggling internal and external priorities with little staff. We have since passed our overdue business records and accounts over to an external Business Manager and Accounts team, an issue we are reassured arises often with overwhelmed new businesses. They have been working over our finances for the last five months, and are still proceeding with a resolution in close sight. We were advised by this team to follow their process and allow them to finalise the donations once all business keepings were accounted first and brought forward.

The article presents that 300,000 downloads have been made, assuming that these were all paid purchases. As most are aware, a small percentage of them had been bringing attention to all the free downloads and promotions we offer in order to make our product and content accessible, our first and foremost priority: accessibility.

TWP is a for-profit company, but has great, enthusiastic intentions of giving back as much as possible to the organisations and charities which the TWP team and community support, respect and are passionate about. The $20,000 we have allocated towards the Asylum Seeker Resource Centre and $2,790 from what *The Age*, refer to as a 'Mothers Day Campaign' to Bumi Sehat Foundation (previously intended to be split with 2h Foundation) hasn't been absorbed by anyone, or TWP, but rather had been accounted for but not processed as per advice.

Though openly discussed with *The Age*, they chose to leave out donations from a private event we held in December 2013 which were handed over to a family with an unwell child, a family put forward by the online community of The Whole Pantry and another in 2013. TWP have made private donations to ASRC which have been receipted and the funding filtration system to Kinfolk Café, a not-for-profit café in Melbourne CBD.

Our books are taking longer to bring up to date than anticipated. TWP forecasted income in October 2014 which was not fulfilled, creating cash-flow issues an unforeseen delays on finalising three discussed charitable donations. TWP's new Business Management and Accounts team are working through the workload of bringing the accounts and businesses up to date and all charities have been openly communicated with and are aware of our intentions to uphold this financial support when the necessary keepings of the business are finalised.

This is an issue which will be resolved with added business support.

In summary I would like to strongly reiterate that in addition to thousands of dollars already donated or gifted to worthy causes, published and otherwise, all remaining promised donations and support will be honoured as soon as the finances are in order, something which has been privately communicated over with the remaining published organisations.

Moving forward into 2015/16, as soon as we are presented with our Profit and Loss statements, we will endeavour to communicate our two nominated partners from herein via Facebook and The Whole Pantry website. These relationships and donations will be managed, externally, by those who administer these transactions, regularly and fully understand the formal process. Corporate media have, in this instance, chosen to omit critical information and publish contradictory statements.

We appreciate your support over the last 18 months and continue to put our community first as we find our footing again.

With Regards
The Whole Pantry Team.

Belle Gibson was in damage control. And it seemed to be working. As we watched on from our iPhone screens, the comments that came in were overwhelmingly supportive of Gibson and overwhelmingly critical of *The Age*. Her followers were sure this was all a misunderstanding, and they went on the attack, hurling accusations at the press of insensitivity, of distorting the truth, and of pursuing only beat-ups and takedowns. There were even one or two comments suggesting this was a vicious campaign by two male journalists hell-bent on destroying the reputation of a young, successful woman.

One early Facebook post said: 'Really not surprised by this media outlet. They need to create a "newsworthy" story and it makes me sick that this spin is what they think will create more clicks/generate more income for them! Rather than a beautiful organisation who has chosen to do all these amazing things in communities. Haters gonna hate!'

'Disappointing but not surprising,' another reader wrote. 'Sensationalist journalists are always trying to stir a controversy out of nothing. Hope you get a chance to voice the truth in a fairer forum x.'

In dozens more supportive comments, many Facebook users accepted Gibson's argument that her new company's teething problems were a valid-enough justification for failing to pass on charity money. 'Such negativity,' one said. 'I have purchased the app and not once have I felt I have been cheated, even after this article. Forgive them for being naive and new to a business and wanting to give something back. You can tell Belle is a genuine person and yes with cancer. Give her a break for wanting or needing to step back and take care of herself and spend precious time with her family. Sending positive vibes Belle. Much love xx.'

Then, bit by bit, post by post, that sentiment started to shift. It shifted very slowly. But before long, it was palpable. Some people began to voice a realisation that Gibson's wordy response had, in fact, done very little, if anything at all, to excuse what she had done. 'Surely money pledged to flow direct to charitable purposes through you is completely irrelevant to cash flow?' one commenter proffered.

Minutes later, the floodgates opened: 'Appalling — your organisation not the media,' another said. 'Money for charity doesn't go into cashflow — that is beyond unethical.'

BOB: You have skipped the point in your very long and wordy response. YOU took money from people who GAVE you the money believing it would go to said charities, you FAILED to forward on the money. YOU have kept the money.

THE WHOLE PANTRY — LIVE HEALTHY: Hi Bob, thank you for your concern and comment. We have covered this many times in this thread, reiterating that we haven't absorbed any money which we intend on donating, rather it is being withheld by our accountants, as all outgoings have, until the rest of the companies [sic] finances are brought up to date. Thank you

LULA: This is nothing short of common thievery and I look forward to seeing justice in due course. LIARS. You don't get to fundraise in the name of charity then keep the funds, not under any circumstances.
THE WHOLE PANTRY — LIVE HEALTHY: We haven't kept any funds, we have addressed this above and privately with three charities who our accountants are holding the donations [for] until the old book keeping is brought up to date

MIKE: So perhaps your marketing campaigns should reflect that you will make a contribution to the nominated charity providing the business is cashflow positive. Otherwise isn't it misleading?
THE WHOLE PANTRY — LIVE HEALTHY: Hi Mike, the issue is that the advice we have received is to get the business accounts up to date into the current Financial Year and then proceed with the outgoings. The second issue is that our projections were incorrect and incoming finances to TWP are delayed which affects what we plan to do from herein, including sustaining the app.

CHRIS: Enriching yourselves while falsely pretending to be helping others in need. Stay classy.

Gibson believed she could weather the storm. For several hours, until well past 2.30 am, she stayed logged on and she fought back, vigilantly responding to nearly every post. She was clinging to the idea that if she kept defending, it would all soon pass. But it wouldn't. It only got worse and more vicious by the second. Soon, her Facebook followers noticed she was deleting some of their most critical comments — and they started screenshotting things that were being scrubbed:

FELICITY: I have just written this comment but had it deleted. I don't think The Whole Pantry team should censor concerned customers who are querying exactly how much of a mess your accounts are in if Belle could go on a cruise around the Caribbean in February before all of this has been sorted out? Surely promises should not be made if they can't be kept.

ROWAN: Team TWP are clearly concerned that things aren't looking good for them at this point in time given they feel the need to delete comments they can't explain away.

SARAH: So many comments being deleted.

BEN: Deleting comments, only proves you have something to hide. Shame on you.
THE WHOLE PANTRY — LIVE HEALTHY: We are not deleting any comments unless they are intentionally erroneous or add to the misinformation of this article. Thank you.

Her attempted censorship did not go down well. For many, it only fuelled confirmation that she had something to hide. 'So disillusioned,' a once-devoted follower bemoaned. 'Oh Belle!'

More questions quickly surfaced. The veracity of her whole story was brought under a cloud.

'Wow … she's got cancer people, where is your compassion!' one user wrote.

'Does she?' another replied. 'I am starting to wonder.'

Some on Facebook, such as a user named Brigitte, hurried to denounce the audacity of interrogating a terminal-cancer sufferer. 'I cannot believe you people believe you have a RIGHT to get an update on Belle's health,' she said. 'Paying a few dollars for an app and following someone on social media does not give you a free pass of entry into someone's private life. Did you all go demanding an update on Delta Goodrem or Olivia Newton John's health?'

But, as Gibson kept deleting, the inquiries persisted:

AMANDA: My comments have been deleted.

JUDY: Mine too. I question her diagnosis.

In the modern-day media cycle, news moves quickly. Tens of thousands of online readers had viewed the article on Sunday night, and it was running in the top slots on *The Age* and *The Sydney Morning Herald* websites all through the busy Monday morning peak-hour rush.

At 10.30 am, an email from The Whole Pantry arrived in our inboxes. It was addressed to our editor, and we had been copied in: 'Request for urgent review of published article'.

'Dear Editor,' it began, 'I am writing … to address some factual inaccuracies and erroneous inferences. In light of Belle taking the brunt of this and needing to put her wellbeing first in preparation for upcoming medical commitments, we put this forward on behalf of the company.'

The 1,200-word email laid out the same arguments included in Gibson's responses to our questions, and repeated much of what had been posted in her Sunday-night rebuttal on The Whole Pantry's Facebook page.

'As a result of this irresponsibly presented article Belle has received a huge backlash on social media, including threats and direct abuse,' the email said. 'We strongly urge that the decision be made for the article to either be rewritten with correct representation of all of the facts and above concerns addressed, comprehensively corrected or retracted in full. We urgently await your response to this issue.'

Our editor in chief replied:

Dear 'The Whole Pantry',
We believe the content of the article is not erroneous and see no need for a retraction.

However Nick and Beau are more than willing to discuss the points raised with Belle Gibson.

The story, by now, was being widely picked up by other Australian media channels. The interest was strong. We were asked to prepare a follow-up story as soon as possible.

We focused on the growing backlash against Gibson, opening the door for the first time to questions surrounding her brain-cancer claims. By late afternoon, it was published online:

Comments casting doubt over Ms Gibson's story of cancer survival are also believed to have been deleted. The 26-year-old, who has traded heavily off her story as a young mother treating terminal brain cancer with nutrition and a healthy lifestyle, declined to discuss her health.

The Age, 9 March 2015

That afternoon, the Whole Pantry Facebook account posted an

announcement on its page. Belle Gibson, it said, was returning to conventional cancer treatment, and had made a 'difficult decision' to step down as the manager of the company. 'Belle is struggling with managing the loss of some of those close to her at the moment,' the post said. 'She has been forced to put the health and wellbeing of herself and her family first. Belle is under the professional care of a new conventional team.' The message continued: 'Belle is not coping, and we ask for respect whilst she grieves and awaits her upcoming appointments.'

But the saga was far from over for Belle Gibson. It would only get worse. Much worse. Adding more fuel to the fire, the very next day, *The Australian* newspaper published a remarkable front-page article, headlined: 'Mega-blogger Belle Gibson casts doubt on her own cancer claims'.

It included explosive comments from Gibson herself, in an interview with journalist Richard Guilliatt, saying it was possible her cancers may have been based on a 'misdiagnosis' by a magnetic-therapy team from Germany.

'It's hard to admit that maybe you were wrong,' she said in an interview, adding that she felt 'confused, bordering on humiliated'.

The Australian, 10 March 2015

The Age's legal team, which had initially been reluctant for us to publish comments from several unnamed sources in Gibson's inner circle stating that they didn't buy her cancer claims, now gave us the all-clear. An article to this effect, 'Friends and doctors raise doubts over Healing Belle cancer claims,' went live that day. It contained details of the 'intervention' that Gibson's friends held for her in her beachside apartment in late 2014, where they confronted her about her diagnosis and urged her to come clean.

We had spoken with multiple cancer specialists over the previous week, who all said off-the-record that Gibson's story of surviving malignant brain cancer just didn't add up. One of the country's most prominent neurosurgeons, Andrew Kaye, head of neurosurgery at the Royal Melbourne Hospital, was the only one prepared to speak out. He said it was *extremely unlikely* for a tumour to spread in the way that Gibson had described:

'There is the very occasional case out of many, many thousands that may have a spontaneous regression ... but I have never seen that,' he said. 'I wouldn't believe any of this unless I saw the pathology report with my own eyes and the pathology itself.'

The Age, 10 March 2015

The media had gone into overdrive. And Gibson went to ground. She wiped thousands of posts and photos from The Whole Pantry's social-media accounts in a desperate attempt to erase history from the internet.

We called Clive again, after the first couple of stories had been published. He was under a lot of pressure. The media was camped outside his house, and people were knocking on the door at all hours. He was angry. Clive said there had been death threats. Their home address had been published online, and so had the name of Oli's school.

'I'm sure you've seen the shitstorm of anger that's being stirred up,' Clive said. 'It's just very unsettling. I understand people's anger and their need for some kind of answers, but that's really crossing the line. That's just dangerous, it's irresponsible.'

Clive, again, said his focus was on protecting Oli and Gibson. 'I understand that the media want answers, everybody else wants answers, but that's really not a concern for me at the moment.'

We talked some more. Clive said he wouldn't be making any statement; he didn't want to inflame the situation. He wouldn't say where Gibson was. At that stage, it wasn't clear if she was in Melbourne. We now know she was on her way home from the US, after Apple had dismissed her. At the end of the call, Clive suggested we meet. He told us he would come to our office at Media House, on Collins Street, at 12.15 pm the following day. The next day we waited for him, but he didn't show.

By the end of the week, Gibson had hired a defamation lawyer. She promised to release a statement; however, it would be two months before the public heard from her again. As the stories piled up, Gibson's staunchest allies, her most trusted friends, started asking her blunt questions directly.

'Do you or did you ever have cancer?' one texted her.

'I am completely broken by the whole thing,' Gibson replied. 'My life has been torn apart, have lost my business, my family and son is under attack. I am not advised to discuss facts at the moment, you already know this. We're doing everything we can right now.'

'It's a simple yes or no,' said the friend. 'If it's a no I'll defend you.'

Gibson never responded.

A feeling shared by many of the people who were close to Gibson was that they needed to be firm with her. It was clear that something was very wrong. They told her she had to come clean, and encouraged her to get help. Gibson, though, became increasingly closed off and paranoid. In one of her final posts on her personal Facebook page, under her long-time pseudonym, 'Harry Gibson,' she fired a parting shot at her friends who had betrayed her by speaking to the press.

'At the end of it, it says more about you, and your priorities, than me or the story you'll get paid to tell,' she wrote. 'With love, and before I get bullied to my death, enjoy your contribution to the world, for I know the work my company and its content did changed hundreds of thousands for the better.'

And then, finally, she started purging the few friends she had left. One by one, she blocked them from her accounts. Some were relieved. 'I'm glad she unfriended me because I was scared to distance myself from her,' said one close friend at the time. 'She is very volatile. It was tormenting seeing her put these posts up. It was giving me the creeps.'

13

WHAT PENGUIN KNEW

Rewind six months.

A car pulled up outside the glass tower on Collins Street in Melbourne's Docklands. A young woman walked out of the foyer and onto the busy footpath. She opened the passenger door and got in. Belle Gibson was rattled. 'She was really concerned,' recalled the driver. 'They grilled her. She said it felt like an interrogation.'

It was late September 2014. Gibson's book was one month from going on sale, and Penguin wanted to prep her for the inevitable publicity. Gibson had obliged. She had come into the publisher's head office and sat down in front of a video camera set up on a tripod. The woman leading the interview was Julie Gibbs. Her colleague, Chantelle Sturt, Penguin's publicity manager, and another Penguin employee, were there, too. Gibson was questioned about the holes in her story. The tape ran for 90 minutes.

Julie and her staff were warm and friendly, but their questions were pointed — the kind of questions they said Gibson could expect to be asked when she was promoting her book. Watching the video today, it seems, at times, like an interrogation. Watching it back, it's difficult to understand why lingering questions about Gibson's story didn't derail the entire project.

Gibson sat on an orange chair in front of a black screen, sipping tea. Her long hair was parted in the middle, falling down over her shoulders, and she wore a black blouse with a light-coloured floral print.

'So,' began Julie, who was off-camera, 'what we wanted to do was take you through a bit — and this is just for us this afternoon — take you through a bit of a questions-and-answer session.'

'Mm-hm,' Gibson replied, sweeping her hair behind her ear.

'So that if you are sitting opposite a *Good Weekend* journalist —

'Yeah.'

'— who's asking you quite investigative questions —'

'Yeah.'

'— you're feeling — we want to rehearse some questions with you.'

'Mm-hm.'

'What we suspect might happen now,' Julie continued, 'is that because you are the success story of the moment, you're one of Australia's great success stories at the moment, you know what journalists do, they want to scratch, scratch, scratching away.'

'Well, they already are,' Gibson said, modestly.

'Yeah, exactly, and we're concerned about that,' Julie replied.

'Well, that's what the publicist at Apple also said. It's like, "What story do you want to be?" Do you want to be [a] strong, entrepreneurial, world-changing woman,' said Gibson, finger-counting.

'Yeah.'

'— or do you want to be-ee — cancer story?'

'Yeah.'

'It's like, "I'm sick of the cancer story."'

'Yep.'

'There's enough of that out there now, there's enough of that in the book.' Gibson raised both hands as if she was about to catch a beach ball. 'Let's make a new story.'

Julie told Gibson this was an exercise they ran through with all high-profile authors. They'd compiled everything about her that was on the public record, and would run through some of the things that were likely to come up. This was a dress rehearsal; a safe place where she could get comfortable workshopping answers to questions about her family, her cancer, her life. They didn't want anyone throwing her off her game.

'I'm going to ask you some of these questions, and some of them you won't like,' Julie said, 'but that's OK because it's just us, alright, and we're here to help you.'

Julie said she had questions prepared. She can be heard shuffling papers. 'Oh, my God —' Gibson said, laughing nervously. She took a sip of her tea with both hands. Her gaze, over the rim of the cup, was fixed on the papers Julie was holding.

Julie Gibbs was warned about problems in Belle Gibson's story at least five months before releasing her book, but no one at Penguin, it turned out, had ever sought evidence to support her claims. In May 2014, Julie was sent an email by one of her senior editors, Nicole Abadee, about concerns in the book's draft. They spanned Gibson's personal story, her employment record, her medical history. 'Julie,' she cautioned, 'I think the main thing to warn Belle about is that there are a few "gaps" which journalists might probe.'

Like so many, Julie was enamoured by the young author's story. But these gaps, as the editor called them, were more like craters, and, in a landmark order several months later, they would cost Penguin

Random House dearly. For Penguin Australia's part in the Belle Gibson saga, the publisher paid $30,000. But the bigger blow was the acknowledgements it had to make. On 22 April 2016, Penguin's general counsel, Briony Lewis, signed an undertaking admitting that the statements made by Gibson in *The Whole Pantry* about her health and charitable endeavours had not been substantiated. Penguin failed to check Gibson's age, diagnosis, prognosis, treatments, and fundraising activities. Put simply, it published whatever she said.

In the undertaking, Consumer Affairs wrote it was concerned that *The Whole Pantry* was directed at people who had cancer, to people with a family history of cancer, and to people whose friends and relatives had cancer. These people, it said, were 'unusually susceptible' in that they were predisposed to being influenced by the false statements made in the book. 'Further, Penguin knew that sales of the book would benefit from Belle Gibson's reputation as a cancer survivor,' it said. 'The director of Consumer Affairs Victoria considers that by publishing *The Whole Pantry*, which contained the untrue statements, Penguin engaged in misleading and deceptive conduct.'

On top of the money, Penguin agreed to improve staff training and develop a risk-management checklist for books making health claims. For at least the next three years, it had to include a prominent warning notice in books making claims that alternative, natural, nutritional, or holistic therapies can treat illnesses. The notice must explain that said therapies are not 'evidenced based' or proven to provide any medical benefit.

Julie Gibbs signed a confidentiality agreement, and left Penguin at the end of 2015, a few months after Gibson's story unravelled. Julie would not speak to us for this book.

***

The video that was recorded in Penguin's offices, a year before Julie's departure, can be difficult to interpret. At times, it doesn't sound like Julie is just rehearsing her author; sometimes she presses her for missing details. Julie looks for little things, little checkpoints, in Gibson's story. Where did she seek out alternative therapies? Was it on the internet? How did she pay for them? Did she have a job at the time? She asks Gibson how old she was at a certain point, then doubles back. *How long ago was that?* At the end of the hour-long interview, the camera is left on, recording Gibson while she eats a salad and chats with Julie and her publisher. It runs for another 30 minutes, and the questions continue. Then Julie apologises and switches it off.

Some topics are clearly off-limits in Penguin's practise interview. On questions about her childhood, Gibson spoke about growing up in Brisbane and leaving home at the age of 12 and living with a supervisor from work. Her eyes dart around the room as she talks.

'What primary school did you go to?' Julie asked.

'I don't even feel comfortable talking about [it],' Gibson replied, scrunching her brow.

'Sure, OK. They're going to ask you all this,' Julie said. 'That's why I'm asking you. OK.'

'Yeah.'

'I think,' the Penguin staffer interjected, 'part of what we're trying to prepare you for is that often times there'll be journalists who are like, "Damn it, I want to go and find that information out for myself", and I guess for you to be able to address it when you feel comfortable, rather than having them go off and do their own special investigation of talking to friends or old schoolmates or whatever it might be, I think it's just protecting yourself, so that the source of truth is you.'

'Yeah,' Gibson said, 'and I just say, you know, "All of my education was in Brisbane", you know, and just saying, like, deflecting even.

But I don't want them to know every nitty-gritty detail or, like, "Who was the person who you lived with?" That's a whole another situation and story, and it's just a micro-detail that no one needs to know or is going to remember.'

'You're going to get asked this more, and more and more —,' Julie said.

But then Penguin just left it there. Unanswered.

Julie turned to her author's employment history. Gibson said her first full-time job was in customer service for a food-services company in Brisbane. She said she was eventually asked to open a 'head office for that division' in Western Australia. Gibson said she was transferred to Perth to open the office, train new staff, and establish logistics networks.

'So what was your role?' Julie asked. 'What were you called?'

'I was leading the business-development end of the customer-service department, and that was, you know, their large-scale customer-service management team. I was just restructuring the business to fit, and training all of those staff.'

'Big job,' Julie said.

'Huge.'

'How old were you when you were doing that?' Gibson was asked.

'Seventeen.'

'God, Belle,' Julie said, laughing. 'You're an old soul, that's all I can say. A very old soul.'

'I know.'

'A very old soul.'

Julie asked Gibson when exactly she had moved over to Perth from Brisbane.

'That was 2008,' Gibson replied.

'2008.'

'I think. I don't know — no, it was earlier than that.'

'Right.'

'Yeah, I was seventeen.'

'You were seventeen?'

'Yeah, so that was seven years ago.'

'Yeah.'

'Yeah.'

It was in Perth, Gibson said, where she suffered a stroke. By now, she had a job at a health-insurance company. She said she was on the phone to a customer one day when she fell off her chair.

'[I] went to the doctor's and they said, "You've had a stroke." Then it was about a week later where the cancer diagnosis —'

'So were you in hospital? Julie asked. 'Did they put you in hospital?'

'No. Like, I had a stroke, and they're like, "You've had a stroke, you're fine."'

'Really?'

'Yeah.'

'Did you do lots of tests?'

'Yeah.'

'So, I was in there for the day,' Gibson said. 'I wasn't in there for a long period of time, and then I was diagnosed with cancer, and, yeah, that just very quick domino effect of everything to come, you know, of — I lost a lot of my short-term memory. Like, my whole life started to crumble, and I'd held it together —'

It had been a couple of months since Gibson had posted on Instagram about her cancer spreading to multiple organs; but then she was off again, travelling around the world. Julie explained that her fans might be a bit confused. Perhaps it was time to update them. They agreed that The Whole Pantry community *had a right to know* about Gibson's health.

'So, Belle,' Julie said, gently, 'looking at what you've announced on your social media —'

Gibson took a deep breath and gave a half-smile.

'— You've said that the cancer is now in your blood and your spleen and your brain and your uterus and your liver. That's really — it's serious now, isn't it?'

Gibson's eyes darted to the side. 'Yeah. Um.' Gibson paused. 'I'm going to get tested for ovarian cancer. I no longer have cancer in my uterus. Woo-hoo,' she said, raising both hands in a cheer motion as she turned to face Chantelle and the other woman from Penguin.

'That's great news,' one said. 'When were you told that?'

'Not long ago.'

'That's great news.'

'Yeah, but it still all feels like it sucks down there,' Gibson said. 'So, you know, I've been putting [it] off for a long time — which isn't intentional, it's just the nature of rocking up to appointments late or on the wrong day because I'm forgetful —'

They joked that Gibson needed the Apple smartwatch.

'I need the Apple watch,' Gibson replied. 'I've been putting off getting my ovaries checked because there's something happening there but ... I feel like cancer is just a manifestation of also just ignoring too many things and it just is the final diagnosis, you know. You get headaches, or you get something. You know, like, you get pains in a particular part of the body, you have a stroke. Like, all of these little individual sequence of events, cancer is the final one, you know? It just is what it is now, you know? To me, it's not intimidating. Like, it's a long list to rattle off and, you know —'

'You look really well,' Julie said.

Gibson knew she looked well. But 'not everything is as it seems,' she told Julie and her publisher. Behind the 'perfectly filtered photos', she was suffering. She might break out in a rash, or be bedridden after a series of seizures.

'Right now, I've got a really stabbing pain in my stomach, which I want to crawl to the floor with,' she said, perfectly composed, 'but it's just that we've not been allowed or empowered to talk about it for so long, that all we do see is what media shows us cancer is or what media shows us dying is. And why can't you die gracefully? Why can't you enjoy that?'

'Do you think you're dying?' Julie asked.

'Yeah.'

'You feel like you're dying?'

'Yeah, and I'm fine with that. And it's conflicting for a lot of people. I don't think I'm going to die tomorrow, but my body is dying. Like, of course it is, you know. It might be a really slow 10 years, but parts of me are shutting down and we only see, you know, really traumatic childbirth, really traumatic death, you know, really traumatic car accidents, and everyone handles it differently, but it's also a choice. Like, I don't choose to feel victimised by this.'

'No,' Julie grinned. 'It doesn't sound like you ever have.'

'No,' Gibson said.

'So, will you now reach [out] to your social-media followers and tell them how you are and what's going on?'

'Yeah.' Gibson nodded. 'It's totally on the list for the week.' Gibson leant forward to pick up her cup of tea.

Gibson was asked about her most recent cancer diagnosis. Had she changed her treatment regime?

'Yeah, I have,' Gibson replied, looking down at the floor.

Gibson struggled to explain the details of a new German therapy she said she was receiving.

'How do you take it?' she was asked. 'What is it exactly?'

'Um,' Gibson hesitated, shaking her head and looking up to the ceiling. 'I don't know how I'm going to talk about this. I might have to do some more reading on it.'

She continued.

'But, it's a machine which is like an electronic pulse, pushes into the cells, and I take medicine when that machine is operating on a program. The program … the computer and machine that I'm on runs this program based on my biology and the way that my body operates through my sleep and times of the day. I take medicine, and this program is opening my cells so the medicine can get into them.'

The three women discussed the importance of being able to convey Gibson's understanding of this new treatment: she needed to have a line or two prepared for when she was asked about it.

'Just a line, exactly,' Penguin told her.

'And it could just be,' Gibson said, 'you know, "I still do my regular check-ins with my oncologists and all of the other modalities that I've respected throughout this whole journey, and have taken on, you know, a European cancer protocol as well." Like, I don't know.'

'You could say you're following a non-conventional European cancer protocol,' Julie said. 'You could certainly do that.'

Gibson ran her hand through her hair. 'Yeah.'

14

CORPORATE RISK

The second week in March 2015 was a very bad week for the team at Penguin who worked on *The Whole Pantry*. Emails were circulating throughout the office, and making their way to staff at the organisation's most senior levels, notifying them that journalists were making inquiries about Belle Gibson. This was an unfolding crisis, and, as big companies often do in times like these, Penguin called in a crisis-management specialist to handle the delivery of an extraordinary admission: it had failed to ask Gibson for any documentary proof of her medical condition before publishing her book. Her claims had never been fact-checked.

'We did not feel this was necessary,' Penguin's statement said, 'as *The Whole Pantry* is a collection of food recipes, which Penguin has published in good faith.'

On the first page of *The Whole Pantry*, the second sentence outlines Gibson's diagnosis and decision to dump conventional medicine. Her entire story, her public profile, had been built and marketed on the strength of her claims of healing herself with nutrition. 'We are concerned about the questions raised in recent days,' Penguin's statement advised. 'We'll discuss them with Belle as ultimately only she can answer the questions.'

No one would have been more concerned than Julie Gibbs, the woman who had taken Belle Gibson under her wing. Julie was calling and texting her author, but two days passed before she received a written response. That's a long time without answers when you're under the media spotlight and it's your career on the line.

The email arrived on 10 March. Gibson was out of town. The email was long. Gibson tried to absolve herself of culpability, and decided to lie to Julie about our email exchange with her. She claimed we had apologised to her, and said there had been a misunderstanding. She also claimed that one of the charities had been misquoted. On her health questions, Gibson kept it brief. She told Julie she was scheduled to undergo another surgery very soon, and would not be speaking about her condition publicly until she had recovered. There was no sign of remorse, and no apology. 'Will be in touch once we manage to work further through this,' Gibson said, signing off for the last time. 'Take care, Jewels.'

Julie promptly wrote back, in what would be her final email to Gibson. She told her author that there would be a message waiting in her inbox from Penguin's lawyer. And she should read it. 'The media situation has escalated and this is now out of my hands,' she told Gibson, 'as we have a situation of corporate risk.'

Penguin's crisis PR consultant was a man named Nick Owens, from Sefiani Communications Group. He helped the Penguin team develop three statements to roll out. He advised them to stagger the responses over the coming three days:

Statement one: CURRENT
We are concerned about the issues raised and have sought an

explanation from Ms Gibson. We have no further comment to make at this time.

Statement two: TOMORROW
We have sought an explanation from Ms Gibson regarding recent questions raised about her medical background but are yet to receive a response from her. Pending a satisfactory response to our questions, we are considering our options regarding our commercial relationship with Ms Gibson and The Whole Pantry.

Statement three: FRIDAY
Penguin Books wishes to advise that it has withdrawn The Whole Pantry recipe book from sale indefinitely. This decision is regrettable but necessary as we are yet to receive a response or explanation from Ms Gibson following the serious issues raised in recent days, despite several requests. Penguin Books regrets any inconvenience caused to retailers or members of the public.

Nick knew what Penguin knew. Gibson's explanation about the fundraising drives was inadequate, and documentary evidence of her health claims probably wasn't coming. 'Belle may even face criminal charges,' he told Penguin executives, 'so the quicker Penguin is distanced from her the better. The only caveat to this is whether your other authors will feel you have cut her loose too hastily without due process (that was one of the sensitivities in the Norma Khouri situation), but I would doubt that is the case here?' (Khouri wrote the 2003 bestseller, *Forbidden Love*, purported to be a true story about her best friend's murder in Jordan, which was later revealed to be a literary hoax.)

Despite the gathering tsunami of public outrage in the first days after the scandal broke, something altogether different was happening at Apple. The smartwatch launch featuring Gibson as one of its star developers was just around the corner. But there were no panicked emails. There were no concerns about the 'situation' or the 'corporate risk'. And there was no mention of crisis-management specialists. The Apple staff who worked most closely with Gibson appeared just as supportive of her as ever.

The mysterious Apple official, TC Chan, was sent a link to *The Age* article by one of Gibson's former friends the day after it was published. A couple of hours later, he wrote back. He was defiant, unwavering in his support. TC still believed in Gibson, and parroted her line about the cash-flow problems the business was facing.

'Yes,' he said, '[the] unfortunate article focused on highlighting startup entrepreneurial issues of competing and conflicting goals, dismissive of great work already done or to be done. Worst of all, it compromises the latter. Spoke with Belle earlier and she is pragmatic about this unpleasantness and determined to take forward steps continuing in the work instead of drawing interest to this kind of blind-sightedness.'

The former friend wrote back, warning TC that Gibson was not just lying about donations — she was lying about *everything*. 'I pray for her and everyone involved with this lie,' he cautioned. 'I hope you can see the light on this and do what is right and help her come clean.' The articles kept coming. But TC never replied.

By the third day of news coverage, when *The Australian* revealed that Gibson herself was unsure of her own diagnosis, Apple again was unperturbed. The very morning the article appeared on the newspaper's front page, Apple's public relations manager, Jesse James, emailed Gibson, approving the smartwatch promotional material for The Whole Pantry. 'Hope you're feeling a bit better today lady,' she signed off.

Gibson, meanwhile, was shoring up support closer to home,

telling friends that she still had the backing of the world's most valuable company. She fired off a text to one friend in Melbourne, asking if he had been contacted by the media and telling him about her plan. 'I've been briefed by a lot of people and have the support of Apple,' she told him, 'so it's just letting the storm calm and then proceed.'

'You can't possibly be making it up,' was his response.

'I don't know anyone capable of that,' replied Gibson.

'Has [Apple CEO] Tim Cook spoken to you directly?'

'One of the new VPs,' Gibson said. 'I can't really discuss this over text.'

Gibson was putting on a brave face. But on a piece of paper in Penguin's Melbourne headquarters, someone who worked on Gibson's book scribbled in black pen what appears to be the summary of a phone call with her:

> Belle distraught.
>
> Three charities still to be paid.
>
> Apple say not to speak to media.
>
> Cancer claims — A. say claims aren't part of it as she's not well.
>
> Apple sending her home tomorrow — she thought she would be there all week.
>
> So many incorrect claims.
>
> Told her not to read the articles — she's being briefed by Ap lawyers and PR.
>
> Her illness will continue — she's clearly unwell.

At Penguin, things were moving fast. Camilla Subeathar in Australia emailed publisher Simon & Schuster in the US. The consumer reaction to the scam was gaining traction in the media. There was more pressure than ever for Penguin to take a stand against

Gibson. They might have to cut her loose sooner than expected.

'We are uncertain that we will receive the evidence we need from Belle and as such, are putting contingencies in place,' Camilla told her colleagues in the northern hemisphere. 'This may include withdrawing the book from sale; this may occur ahead of the deadline we have given Belle due to the speed with which the story is moving and the fundamental issue of Belle's credibility.'

It had been less than a week, but the public pressure on Penguin had already reached tipping point. Nick Owens suggested withdrawing the book earlier than planned. 'If you look like you're resolved to do that,' he said, 'from a PR perspective it's worth considering making that announcement today to get on the front foot a little. You may still get questions about how much Penguin knew in advance (which you can decline to respond to).'

Penguin's customers had already begun asking pointed questions:

Do you take all information you are given at face value? I believe you should hold up on all her publishing and PR until this has been thoroughly checked by the police.

Normally I'm not a keyboard warrior, but this author lied about serious illness in order to build a business that ultimately led to your company publishing her book. If Penguin has any type of ethical procedures, this is surely the time to take action and ban this book from further print runs and current sales.

If you go ahead with her book, you have just as much blood on your hands as she does. Supporting someone who faked terminal cancer to dangerously influence true sufferers to not utilise scientifically proven medicine is not illegal, but my god is it unethical.

We find it absolutely appalling that Penguin is still publicising (and selling) the subject book on its website. How can a respected publisher like Penguin, with all conscience, continue to support the fraud, liar and, worst of all, charity stealing con artist that Belle Gibson has been exposed as being.

I request a full refund for my fraudulent purchase. My transaction supported the fabricated lies, while there are individuals suffering each day with cancer who struggle to pay for their treatment. The thought of my money profiting this scam is disgusting!

I have cancer all around me and to hear what this woman may have done is despicable. As a publishing house, do you not have an obligation to your readers that what you are promoting is true? I would like a refund for this book as I don't believe anyone should be making money from this.

And this, from a woman who said her husband died from brain cancer, aged 51:

[It] sickens me to the core any human could lie regarding a terminal illness when so many people this day and age are struck down with cancer. It's the treatment, it's the hope, it's praying for a cure, it's trying anything and everything to keep the cancer at bay. To this day I am so proud of my late husband for his courage and his spirit will live forever in my heart. As for Belle Gibson I have no compassion for her at all, and I just feel for the innocent people that purchased her book living in hope that they too could cure their terminal illness.

Penguin's letter arrived at Gibson's townhouse by registered mail on 16 March. But she didn't open it. Perhaps, by now, the gravity of the situation had finally sunk in. It was all over. The book was being pulled. Her overseas publishers, the Penguin Random House-owned Michael Joseph in the UK, and Atria, a division of Simon & Schuster in the US, would cancel their upcoming launches. Victoria's consumer watchdog opened an investigation into The Whole Pantry, one that would ultimately land her in the Federal Court of Australia.

But for Gibson, the worst was still yet to come. Apple was working with her in secret in the US on the smartwatch. It had planned an exciting announcement at the launch, but the young mother and her app were notably absent from the proceedings. It had taken a week, but, finally, inside Apple, there was a flurry of emails about the young Australian woman who had been picked from millions. The news reverberated back to its headquarters in California, with executives including the senior public relations manager, Ted Miller, being notified. Luke Bevans, the Australia and New Zealand App Store manager, emailed Matt Fischer, the vice president of the App Store, in the US as the coverage entered its second week. 'Last week the story started breaking via Fairfax Media,' he wrote. 'And so the backlash started, and snowballed over the last week, with front page headlines, resulting in the book deal being scrapped and our removal from featuring today.'

'[TC Chan] has had a close relationship with Belle and was in Cupertino last week dealing with ANZ developers in the Watch Lab, as well as talking to her. TC and PR informed me yesterday that Belle is waiting for this to blow over and is taking legal advice, but this morning that may have changed. When we hear from her we'll let you know. The story is now a full national news story, and our removal of featuring will be commented on.'

By the following morning, Tuesday 17 March, The Whole Pantry app was being pulled from all Apple platforms. Its online promotions were wiped from the Apple website. Then it disappeared from the

App Store. Gibson's first corporate supporter, and most high-profile partner, had silently severed all ties with her.

Apple said nothing. It rarely makes comments in the media, but this was a case in which the public demanded and expected an explanation. Apple's approach was simple: ignore questions, and don't give the story any more oxygen. In conversations with journalists at the time, on background, Apple's PR staff attempted to distance the company from Gibson by painting its relationship as strictly professional. Gibson was an app developer, just like any other, Apple claimed. However, the relationship was anything but. The best way to describe it would be chummy: Gibson was wholly embraced by senior staff.

Time and again, Apple published false statements about Gibson being diagnosed with cancer, eschewing conventional medicine, and embarking on a quest to heal herself naturally. But never once did anyone at the company make any inquiries about these claims. No one questioned her. Instead, Apple said it relied on the information Gibson provided and that its app testing was limited to technical functionality and compliance with developer policies. The tech giant would later tell an Australian court that The Whole Pantry was withdrawn from sale in March 2015 due to a 'lack of compliance' with its policies:

> Around this time Apple Australia became aware through the press of false statements made by the developer about her medical condition and also that she was donating to charity (but was not). Ms Gibson was expected to respond back to the App Store review team. She did not, and her app was never reinstated.

Today, Apple refuses to speak Gibson's name. Never before has the company so publicly embraced a new talent and then cut him or her loose without uttering a word. And it has never released a statement about its partnership with Belle Gibson.

'In relation to your story,' wrote Fiona Martin, Apple's director of communications, 'we have nothing further to add.'

Around the world, all who had befriended, worked with, or endorsed Belle Gibson were wiping their hands of her. Included among them was American food-and-beverage public relations firm, YC Media, a high-profile agency that has worked on campaigns for some of the world's most famous chefs. With Jamie Oliver, Ferran Adria, Emeril Lagasse, Curtis Stone, Cat Cora, and the Voltaggio Brothers on its client list, the firm had been hired to promote the 2012 centenary of the birth of Julia Child, widely regarded as the first-ever celebrity chef. It had also been picked to run a three-month campaign to promote Gibson's US book launch. A flattering black-and-white photograph of Gibson, laughing, graced the client page on its website until around the middle of March, when someone in the New York office logged on to their computer and deleted it.

-15-

YOU DON'T LIE ABOUT CANCER

In the space of one week, Belle Gibson had gone from being universally adored to being wholly despised. One commentator characterised the phenomenon as a Full Sympathy Reversal, in which 'every ounce of goodwill directed her way ... has now been recast as rage and contempt.'

One fan wrote: 'I bought your app. I bought your cookbook. I read about you in *Marie Claire*. I watched you on various TV shows. I followed you on Instagram. I rooted for you and felt sad for you when you posted about your cancer spreading. And now I am just appalled.'

Said another: 'I'm still in shock. I downloaded her app, and followed her on Instagram. When she broke the news her cancer spread all over I shed some tears. Why? Because I lived that pain through my family members who died like that. I feel so hurt that she would take advantage of something so devastating like cancer.'

'I admired her and loved her,' said one person who was close to Gibson. 'Now I feel like an idiot.'

Revelations that Gibson had kept money raised for charity and appeared to be lying about having cancer ignited a furious response. In the newsroom, we were inundated with emails from readers. Never before had we received such an overwhelming reaction to a story we'd written. Doctors, nurses, and cancer patients came forward. So did parents of children with cancer, children of parents with cancer, friends of people with cancer, people who work for charities, people who downloaded the app, people who had bought the book, and people who were just really pissed off.

They united with thousands of others online against what our society considers an unforgivable lie. Their messages didn't just attack Gibson; they slammed Apple and Penguin for their part in the scandal, for giving her a platform, for lending credibility to her story, and for validating it. People pledged to boycott both companies, and demanded refunds for the app and book. The con had touched a deeper vein. Gibson's deceit affected not just her followers, but people who had never even heard of her previously:

I have read your story about this woman who appears to be masquerading as a cancer survivor for financial gain. As a cancer survivor, such behaviour appals me, to say the least. I survived stage 3 rectal cancer in 2008 and then throat cancer in 2012. I would love to come face to face with this woman to confront her with the terrible pain and suffering that genuine cancer patients endure, often with fatal outcomes.

Doesn't she comprehend that there will be people out there that will take her advice hoping they get control or cure their cancer. She could be accountable for lives that are lost because they read her articles about how she healed herself. Indirectly her voice could destroy lives.

Never in eight years of being a consultant radiologist have I ever heard or seen of a 'terminal (in 4 months) primary brain cancer' spreading to any organ other than the brain or spine. I have very serious doubts as to the validity of her claims.

I am furious and sickened by what Belle Gibson got away with, and in despair that she has faced no punishment whatsoever. [The] Australian Competition and Consumer Commission and Victoria Police should be all over such an obvious fraud and thief. Instead she has made a mockery of the laws and conventions designed to prevent this type of exploitation.

I am very concerned that Penguin books still appear to be shortly releasing Belle Gibson's in the US/UK. Surely given the issues raised it is, at the very least, immoral to release a book that may be proven to have been based on lies. I am also concerned that potentially millions of Apple watch customers will also unknowingly be adopting practices that may well be based on a fraudulent business.

As someone who works in the not-for-profit sector and relies on the faith and goodwill of the public for funding, I applaud your investigation into The Whole Pantry. I am also a cancer survivor and find the whole story troubling.

Please don't let this story die. Frauds like this deserve to [be] chased to the end of the earth. I don't know her but find pretending to have cancer to claim sympathy and obtain profit just so wrong.

***

There was a knock at the door. Penne and Wolfgang Schwarz had a sense of foreboding that it wasn't good. They had already started to feel like outsiders in their neighbourhood; they had noticed the glares in the supermarket aisles, and heard the whispers at school. And now, finally, their community was on their doorstep. Penne and Wolfgang let them in. What their neighbours wanted was proof — proof that their son, Joshua, five, was dying.

The Schwarzes lived in the Dandenong Ranges, about 40 minutes to the east of Melbourne. It's semi-rural territory; the type of place where people are close, where neighbours know each other. In 2013, Penne started telling people that Joshua had been diagnosed with terminal brain cancer, that he had been given four months to live. There was no treatment to save Joshua — Joshy, as the family call him. His cancer, an anaplastic astrocytoma, grade three, was caused by a rare genetic disorder, and it was incurable.

There was an immediate and spontaneous outpouring of support. The close-knit community banded together and rallied around the family: they organised fundraisers in Joshua's name, there were food drives, and offers of practical help around the Schwarzes' house. The local newspaper and television station both covered the little boy's story.

Joshua outlived the four-month prognosis given by doctors. And, by Christmas, people started to ask questions. All of a sudden, there were doubts, and those doubts soon infected the small community. What had happened to the fundraising money? Why were his parents renovating their house? Why hasn't Joshua lost his curly brown hair? Why was he still at school? Did he even have cancer?

Joshua was sidelined, excluded from playing with other children. Penne was confronted in the street more than once. By the time their neighbours showed up on her doorstep, Penne was at breaking point. She'd already fallen out with many people in the area.

Even though he knew the answer, Wolfgang asked why they were there. They weren't going to stop until they saw evidence that his son was going to die. 'When my husband asked them what is it that they wanted, they said a funeral would have been good. That's the point I broke down,' Penne recalls, through tears. 'One of the women said, "Look, I know it sounds horrible, but that's what people were expecting, and when it didn't happen people became suspicious."' The Schwarzes handed over a letter from Joshua's oncologist, and copies of MRI brain scans. And then the neighbours left.

We spoke to half a dozen of the people in Penne's community who were sceptical about Joshua's cancer diagnosis. A couple of them steadfastly believed his parents were faking the illness the whole time, while others believed they overstated their son's condition. 'He's still alive,' said one. 'No money, from what I can tell, has gone to Joshua's treatment.' Another admitted, 'I'm one of quite a few people wondering what's going on with the money [they] received. He hasn't missed much school at all, and always seems to be in good health.' One woman said, 'They maintain that the treatment was very successful. If that's the truth, then it was.'

Those who doubted Joshua's diagnosis had many unanswered questions about what happened to the money — the tens of thousands of dollars — that was raised. They believed it was going to be put towards overseas medical treatment, but claim, without any proof, that the family used it instead to renovate their house and go on holidays. 'I'm quite sure that it is a scam,' one said. 'They drive around in two four-wheel-drives, really nice cars. If [Joshua] has got 16 weeks to live and no money, wouldn't you sell at least one of them?'

Penne called us a couple of days after Gibson was exposed. She knew the social-media star personally; they were friends after having been introduced on social media. Joshua and his father had attended

Oli's fourth birthday party, and Gibson's family had been invited to their home. Their kids played together. In the back of her book, Gibson acknowledges Penne and Joshua. To Penne, she writes: 'Here is a printed invitation to my love and support.' She calls Joshua 'the second little man after my own heart' and the person with whom she shares 'an unintimidated friendship with our "brain bugs".' In January 2014, Gibson was among hundreds of people to attend a local fundraiser for Joshua. The event was held just weeks after she had written on Instagram that 100 per cent of app sales for a week would be donated to the family.

Gibson's post about fundraising to support Joshua was revealing:

Josh has a similar malignant, inoperable brain tumour to the one I have. From the greatest ache and pains in my heart, I feel this little boy's journey and story. Like I said last night — for the week, we chose to this family to donate 100 per cent of app sales to, in hopes to find them a medicine, holistic or happy miracle. If you've already bought the app, you can go to the link in my profile and buy a 'virtual ticket' to our world changing events — this 'ticket' (donation) gives you power to give back to those without support, inspiration, education or the quality of life most of us are blessed with every day.

The virtual ticket related to Gibson's first-ever fundraiser. The Schwarz family was one of four beneficiaries promoted. Gibson claims to have given the family money in cash. But Penne said she knew nothing of the fundraising drives in her youngest child's name, and that her family had never received a cent from Gibson. The Federal Court of Australia agreed with Penne.

One of Gibson's friends, Chanelle, remembers being asked by her, in 2014, to organise meals for the Schwarz family. Chanelle said she spent two days cooking, and delivered them to Gibson's home. 'About a week later, she told me she delivered all of the meals to them,' the friend said. 'Months later, I found nearly all of the meals stacked in her freezer.'

Penne contacted us to ask a question. She wondered if Gibson might have become close to her to model her story off that of her little boy, to make hers more believable. We told her what we knew — it seemed unlikely. Gibson never sought out the Schwarz family. A mutual friend had introduced them. And Gibson, by the time she met Josh, had already been faking cancer for years. Penne says she never had any reason to doubt Gibson's story, but like the young woman's other new friends, she had never previously been told a great deal about Gibson's past.

In those first days after Gibson was exposed, Penne felt that she had been exploited by Gibson, that her son had been used. She called Gibson to ask if the story was true. 'She avoided directly answering anything that I was asking her,' Penne said. 'She was deflecting it onto how difficult this was on her, and how she needed to focus on her own health. She didn't address anything that I was raising with her.'

Penne was upset and cried through much of our phone call. But she wanted to impress on us that, despite what Gibson had done, she needed support. Lynching her was not the answer. After all, she had been through it. 'I can kind of relate with some parts of what's happening to Belle because we've been down a similar path [under] very different circumstances,' she said. 'Joshua didn't die when he was supposed to, so there was a backlash in the community.

'It's been atrocious. People became suspicious of our family. One mother said, "If he really has cancer, why does he still have hair?" When people fundraise for you, it's like they're invested. I had one lady come up to me in the street and ask me about the money. She felt that she had the right to question everything, that he had become public property.'

On 21 January 2017, Joshua died. He was nine years old.

The messages from cancer patients and their families kept coming:

> As a cancer survivor, it has meant the world to me to have this perspective brought to light. I started following @healing_belle just as her star was rising. I fell for Belle Gibson's story hard. I most resonated with her because of her posts on cancer. I was going through something I didn't know how to talk about, what language to use, I didn't even tell anyone I worked with I had cancer — I just took leave. And here was this girl, so much braver than I, telling the world her story and inspiring people like me. I even remember scrolling through her feed in my hospital bed the day after my surgery, looking for inspiration and hope from someone who'd been there and knew how much it sucked. I wished I could be as strong as her, to heal myself with food and a natural approach but I was scared. Everything moved so quickly and I had a fundamental faith in science & medicine that propelled me to jump into treatment within 24 hrs of diagnosis. Nonetheless, it was a tremendously tumultuous year where I doubted myself and my choices, especially compared to the sexy, modern and all natural cancer-fighting style of Jess Ainscough and Belle Gibson. It was rare to see cancer icons that were my own age and were full of life despite their diagnoses. That's something big for me: I downloaded her app at first chance, I told my mom, friends, shopkeeper to get it too, I purchased all her holiday pack upgrades, posted solidarity Instagrams dedicated to her when her health took a turn, made her recipes and actively participated in #thewholepantry community. I even paid double to

have her book shipped overseas from Australia because I couldn't wait for the wider release.

And:

My daughter has Hodgkin's Lymphoma, and has heeded the calls of this fraud to pay for her apps, follow her fraudulent path, and risk death. As a medical general practitioner, I can only offer rational treatment. It is impossible, in any philosophical debate, to prove that a negative is wrong, so my daughter flew with the belief that an unproved positive must be right.

And:

I am just so disgusted. I have two children with chronic illness (not cancer) and it is so hard to get funding and understanding. I bought her app and book for my 17 year old daughter who is ill. She today is disgusted and deflated that we were misled by someone who has preyed on vulnerable sick people. Karma will find her I believe.

One woman, Heather, told us how she and her husband had flown into Melbourne from Adelaide to be with their 31-year-old daughter, Jane, when she was diagnosed with cancer. Jane had gone for a scan after complaining of abdominal pain, and a tumour was found in her ovary. The surgeons cut it out and put it on the scales: it weighed 1.4 kilograms. At first, the cancer, which is called a mucinous adenocarcinoma, was thought to be metastatic. Doctors told the family there was a 97 per cent chance it was a secondary cancer from the small bowel or pancreas. That is, there was a 97 per cent chance it was terminal.

Heather said it was while waiting for the results that she realised there was nothing she would not do to save her daughter.

'Your house, possessions, your own life, anything,' Heather said. 'But sometimes all you can give is hope and support, and this should come from family, friends, the medical profession, and people who have experienced at first hand the treatment and aftermath of a malignant diagnosis. There are a lot of stories of hope out there, and that is what people like my daughter need to hear — real positive stories, not false hope spread by charlatans the like of Belle Gibson.'

After a series of tests and a six-week wait, the family learned that Jane's cancer was, in fact, a primary. She was in the lucky 3 per cent, and would go on to have a healthy son with the help of IVF. In the future, she will need to have more surgery, and, eventually, a hysterectomy. But she has a much better chance of survival than first thought.

Heather remembers Jane telling her about Belle Gibson, whom she had met in Melbourne, and about the new app she had downloaded. For a long time, Gibson made her angry. 'She profited from offering false hope to people who are enduring genuine illness,' Heather said. 'There are lots of children and young adults who are having to cope with cancer, and quite a lot of positive stories as a result of medical and surgical intervention, with no harm in complementary therapies, healthy diet, and lifestyle.'

'But,' said Heather, 'you don't cure a brain tumour or any other malignant tumour in your pantry cupboard.'

Another woman, from Melbourne, wrote to us asking if we knew how she could get a refund for the two books and the app that she bought. She told of the faith she had placed in Gibson's story: she said every week she and her sister would spend hours trawling the city's markets to track down the ingredients listed in *The Whole*

Pantry cookbook so that they could prepare the nutritious meals for their father, who had terminal lung cancer. Although she knew he could not be cured, she told us she was heavily invested in Gibson's story, and hoped that following her regime might buy her dad more time.

It didn't. 'I had faith in this lady's story and implemented some things with my father who passed away last week from cancer,' she wrote. 'Now to read her story has no truth to it is very heart breaking and [an] absolute disgrace to her.' The woman's father died earlier than doctors had expected, the week before the Gibson scandal broke, in March 2015.

Sydney doctor Lester Pepingco penned Gibson an open letter, warning about the danger of the *miracle cure* she was peddling:

Dear Belle Gibson,

I'm a medical doctor. I currently work in general practice after seven years of university and then five years of postgraduate training in hospitals and clinics, with one more year to go. While working in Royal Prince Alfred Hospital as a resident, I did a term in medical oncology. This term was eye opening and completely changed my view of non-evidence based placebo therapy.

During that awful residency term in medical oncology, I saw the devastation which can occur out of the desperation of a terminal illness. I saw this desperation lead to families travelling overseas to abandon evidence-based medical treatments in favour of expensive therapies which involved everything from curing malignancies with herbs and juices to another patient travelling overseas to be wrapped in tinfoil and placed in a bath out in the sunlight. I witnessed [a] patient with metastatic malignancy take long haul flights overseas to China after being offered a cure by 'natural healers'. Upon their return, the malignancy had not only progressed due to the interruption of their chemotherapy but the patient also developed a devastating deep vein thrombosis and pulmonary embolism which is a complication secondary to a combination of their malignancy coupled with the long haul flight.

These mind-boggling and often bizarre treatments all share two very common traits. Firstly, they are incredibly expensive. I remember one family placing themselves into catastrophic debt months before their primary breadwinner was to now pass away. Secondly, these treatments are based on the always anecdotal 'one girl had cancer and she took these herbs and now she doesn't'.

Sound familiar?

Belle Gibson, you are that 'one girl'. When you so irresponsibly misconstrue and advertise your story of cancer survival, it creates a deception with real consequences on the lives of other people and their families. Your story creates a false hope which causes patients to abandon therapies with demonstrated efficacy in favour of ridiculous and dangerous placebo treatments.

[The late] Sam de Brito wrote an article last week about the 'wellness warrior', Jessica Ainscough who after being diagnosed with cancer, flouted conventional medical treatments in order to 'conquer cancer with carrot juice'. The outcome? She passed away at the age of 30. Prior to that, her own mother was diagnosed with breast cancer and again refused conventional medicine and chose the same therapy.

Cancer can be a devastating disease. It can rob people of their dignity and render them completely vulnerable. We should do our utmost to support them out of this vulnerability instead of taking advantage of it for profit.

Kind regards,
Lester Pepingco

The public, and then Gibson's fans, rounded on her. Her home address was published on the internet, and Gibson is said to have received death threats. Hundreds of vicious comments directed at The Whole Pantry founder detailed her devotees' feelings of betrayal and heartbreak. The staff and the few friends that Gibson had left abandoned her. A new Facebook page, *Belle Gibson Uncovered*, sprung up online, collating all the news coverage, and attracting thousands of angry followers almost overnight.

The rage was amplified by Gibson's silence, her refusal to speak out, to defend herself, to offer an explanation, to apologise, in the face of growing anger that she had traded off the fake story of cancer survival to build her global brand.

ADMISSIONS

Sometime towards the end of March, Alex Twomey answered his mobile. It was an old friend with a strange favour to ask. It was to do with someone he had never heard of.

'Do you know Belle Gibson?'

Gibson had been all over the news lately, and Alex was quite the consumer of news: he was, after all, a media adviser. But his clients were large corporations, market-listed companies. He didn't have an Instagram account, he didn't follow any wellness bloggers, and he wasn't much into dieting. He scrunched his brow and thought for a bit longer. Nope. He had never heard of her.

'Who is she?' he asked.

The caller explained that Gibson was a friend of a friend, and she was in a whole world of trouble. She had told everyone she had cancer and, now, it certainly seemed, this wasn't the case.

'She doesn't know anyone,' the caller said. 'All the media are just hounding her. She doesn't know what to do.'

'Is she claiming this is all a big misunderstanding,' Alex asked, 'or is it all true and she wants to confess?'

'She wants to confess. But she doesn't know who to.'

Although at first hesitant, Alex ultimately agreed. It wouldn't be a huge job. And if she was ready to come clean, hers was an important story about false hope and miracle cures that had to be told. He said he would meet with Gibson and put her in touch with someone who would tell it. His old friend said she would really appreciate that. They hung up, and Alex went back to his usual work, unaware that his career was about to take a very strange detour.

In March 2015, Alex was the managing director of Bespoke Approach, a boutique but big-name corporate advisory firm, founded by two former federal MPs, a political lobbyist named Ian Smith and another named Andrew Butcher, who had been senior vice president for News Corp in New York City, and a long-time confidant to Rupert Murdoch.

Alex is the opposite of the silver-tongued PR guy. In his early 40s, he is down-to-earth, mellow-mannered, and genuinely funny. For the better part of the past decade, he has worked in corporate public affairs, sometimes as a spokesman, but far more often he was the man behind the scenes — a crisis manager, or what's often more tactfully called an *issues* manager. His job was to give advice to company boards running the nation's largest builders, miners, insurers, and retailers, especially when they found themselves in thorny situations. Bespoke Approach was a small firm with big clients, and offices in two cities. Its offices in Melbourne were inside an elegant and narrow-fronted brick building at the top end of Flinders Lane.

Belle Gibson arrived at the meeting alone. She walked up the skinny stairway and introduced herself to Alex. 'Thanks for meeting with me,' the young woman said. 'I've got myself into terrible trouble.' Gibson was shown into a room, and she sat down and started talking. Right from the start, her story was vague. Too vague and too fluid, Alex recalls, and she choked on tears the whole way through telling it. Whenever he tried to drill her down on the countless gaps in key parts of her storyline, she would simply say, 'I can't remember.' She told Alex she felt like an idiot, and claimed that she herself had been taken for a ride by alternative therapists. Alex sat and listened, trying to make sense of what he was hearing. He tried, at times, to give her the benefit of the doubt, but he struggled to believe most of what she was saying. One thing was clear to him: 'This was not a super-bright kid.'

He asked her if she could provide proof — any proof at all — that she had been misdiagnosed, and Gibson presented some paperwork. They appeared to be the results of some strange electromagnetic tests that had been conducted at a naturopathic centre near Wollongong, in New South Wales. They *looked* like medical reports — they contained a table titled 'patient data' and what purported to be images of various cells — but they were nothing of the sort. At the bottom of each page was a sentence advising that the report 'should not be used to diagnose any medical condition'. The word 'cancer' was not mentioned anywhere, but it didn't take Alex long to form the view that some so-called practitioners in this unregulated world of 'alternative wellness', or whatever you wanted to call it, had at least lent a degree of credibility to Gibson's bogus belief that she was sick. 'I couldn't believe these guys existed,' Alex recalls, shaking his head incredulously. 'Maybe on some level she did think she was sick.' But, still, there was nothing that could corroborate any of her elaborate claims of a cancer diagnosis, of ditching chemotherapy, or of ever visiting a hospital, which she had used to build her brand. And whatever way you sliced it, Alex believed, Gibson was culpable, and 'she was going to cop it'.

Was she an out-and-out fraud? Or was she a compulsive liar, a naive kid, who had let a bogus story run away from her, perhaps even partly believed it at times, and somehow found herself in the happy position of being presented with the opportunity of a lifetime? Alex was left convinced of the latter. If it was a highly calculated scam, he thought, it certainly wasn't a sophisticated one.

'I don't know what to do,' Gibson sobbed over and over. 'I've wrecked everything.'

In his role as a corporate media adviser, one of the most significant parts of Alex's job was to tell it straight, to give the brutal, honest truth, to powerful executives who weren't used to hearing it, and who may not have wanted to hear it. The advice he gave Gibson that morning, not surprisingly, was just as frank. He told her to come clean, to tell her story publicly, to settle any debts, and disappear somewhere.

'Go to a country town. Change your name. And disappear.'

This made Gibson cry even more. 'Do you think there is any way of bringing back the business?' she asked him.

'No,' he told her, gently but straightforwardly. He recalls that Gibson really didn't seem to get it. 'You're done ... You lied to people about having cancer. The best you can hope for is to stop the media coming after you. And at least once you tell your story, there's not going to be a whole lot left.'

That night, in something of a complete coincidence, Alex attended a function at Eureka Tower, a 91-storey skyscraper in Melbourne's Southbank district, and bumped into Helen McCabe. Helen was the editor-in-chief of the *Australian Women's Weekly*, the nation's best-known glossy women's magazine. By now, Belle Gibson was the hottest story in town. News of her charity fraud, and accusations that she had lied about cancer, had been picked up by just about every major media outlet in the country. Stories like this one don't come up every day. *This is a bit of fate*, Alex thought, as he approached Helen, with an offer for the exclusive. The *Weekly* was perhaps the best option for Gibson's tell-all. It had a focus on long-form profile stories and current-affairs features. It was a national publication, with more than 1.5 million readers, so Gibson couldn't be accused of hiding. It would be a sit-down and in-depth interview, but not a live broadcast. Gibson's story was too sloppy for TV or radio, Alex thought. There was too much potential for disaster with that.

'She was hot media property,' was the view of Bryce Corbett, the magazine's chief of staff at the time. 'Everyone wanted Belle Gibson.'

Helen McCabe leapt at the offer, and they set the wheels in motion. Bryce Corbett assigned the story to Clair Weaver, an experienced reporter based at their Sydney newsroom. Clair was no puff-piece journo. She had recently shot to national attention for revealing health officials' concerns around the potentially deadly impact of Pete Evans' 'baby paleo' diet, and she has written at length about the perils of the wellness and anti-vaccination movements. Clair flew down from Sydney. There were two interviews with Gibson, face-to-face, in Bespoke's Melbourne offices. Alex sat in on them both, but only as an observer.

Gibson had her hair in a neat ponytail, and wore a cream shirt and jeans. Clair recorded the interviews, and later played them back to Bryce. He was left feeling the same as Alex had after his first meeting with her.

'Her testimony was mercurial,' Bryce says. 'You could never, at any point, pin her down. She'd say something, and you'd go to pin it down — whether it was a date or a name of somebody — and she'd sort of backtrack and change the story. She was really reluctant to commit to anything or any part of her story. She wanted to keep it all fluid. You didn't know whether she was a master manipulator or whether you were supposed to feel sorry for her because she has this problem where she is some sort of compulsive liar.'

In the days before publication, Alex received the odd call from Clair, checking certain details, 'just the normal post-interview mopping up'. He also received occasional calls from Gibson. He encouraged her to lay low.

In late April 2015, the article appeared. Gibson's photo was on the front cover, next to the headline, 'The Girl Who Conned Us All'. A two-page spread ran inside, under the headline, 'My Lifelong Struggle with the Truth':

Belle Gibson claimed to be healing her terminal cancer with wholefoods — but now it's proven to be a cruel web of lies. Yet is Belle a hoax mastermind or simply troubled?

FRESH-FACED. Earnest. Naive. When Belle Gibson speaks, she cries easily and muddles her words. She's passionate about avoiding gluten, dairy and coffee, but doesn't really understand how cancer works. All of which begs the question: is this young woman really capable of masterminding one of the biggest hoaxes in recent history?

This is the pretty 23-year-old who convinced millions of people she was miraculously healing her terminal brain cancer through healthy eating and natural therapies. The mother-of-one's 'inspirational' story was going global — with her wellness app, *The Whole Pantry*, handpicked by US giant Apple for its new smartwatch and her cookbook scheduled for release in America and the UK — when it all began to unravel.

Surely, you might assume, this is evidence of someone with street smarts? Former friends take it further, dubbing her 'manipulative', 'a sociopath' and 'a wolf in sheep's clothing'. The truth, however, is more complicated.

In two lengthy interviews with *The Weekly* this month, it seems that sometimes even Belle is unsure where the truth ends and the fantasy begins.

'I am still jumping between what I think I know and what is reality,' she tells *The Weekly*. 'I have lived it and I'm not really there yet.'

Later in the piece, there it was. Gibson's long-awaited admission:

The Weekly asks Belle outright if she has or ever has had cancer.

'No,' she confesses. 'None of it's true.'

And how did it feel, after more than five years of claiming she was terminally ill, when she confronted this truth?

'It's just very scary, to be honest,' she says, her voice wobbling. 'Because you start to doubt the crux of things that make up who you are. You know, I'm blonde and I'm tall, and I've got hazel eyes and I've got cancer. And all of a sudden, you take away some of those high-level things and it's really daunting.'

Alex Twomey's phone blew up. He hadn't known he was going to be named in the piece, but he had been. The morning *The Weekly* came off the presses, he found himself inundated with calls and emails from journalists wanting their one-on-one with the woman who had fooled the world. Gibson called him, too. But because of all the crying, she was hard to hear down the line. 'She was in tears,' Alex recalls, 'very distressed, saying how harsh and hard to read it was.'

The Weekly's big scoop soon went viral. It made headlines worldwide — headlines that usually contained one quote that said it all: 'No, None of it is True'. BBC News ran with the story. So did *Cosmopolitan*, the UK's *Daily Mirror*, *The Washington Post*, *The Irish Times*, *VICE*, and Canada's *Globe* and *Mail*.

Bryce took several phone calls from Gibson in the days that

followed. She was extremely distressed about how the article had turned out. 'How *else* did she think it was it going to turn out?' Bryce wondered. In one conversation, he recalls, Gibson kept saying she couldn't understand why everyone was being so awful to her. 'What about all the people I helped?' Bryce remembers her asking, or about the app she'd built that had 'so many positive contributions to people's lives?' She couldn't understand why everyone was so focused on the cancer diagnosis. She had believed it to be true.

In one part of the article, the *Weekly* had also raised the question of whether Gibson might have been afflicted with what's known as Munchausen syndrome — a mental disorder in which someone fakes an illness to gain sympathy and attention:

> So what causes someone to develop a disorder like this? Dr Melissa Keogh, a clinical psychologist in Melbourne, says, 'Often there will be an underlying personality disorder and history of early childhood trauma. Compulsive lying tends to be associated with more severe personality disorders. With narcissistic personality disorder, people see themselves as superior. They will lie to get what they want because they think they are entitled to do so. They want to be adored by other people, so they will try to get attention whenever they can. People with borderline personality disorder strongly fear abandonment or being seen in a negative way by other people, and mistruths in this case are often desperate attempts to avoid these situations.

'Belle was really upset about that,' Bryce recalls, 'really upset that there was any suggestion there was something wrong with her mentally. She was affronted.

'It would have been like pleading insanity on a murder charge, and, in some respect, it would have been the easy way out ... but she was determined for that not to be the case. She was determined to be painted as the victim in all of this.

'There was a certain amount of delusion.'

On one of his phone calls with Gibson, Alex tried to remind her that she *knew* it was going to be like this; she was told that it would be bad. She had admitted taking people's money by using the myth of having cancer. There was no scenario — not now, not ever — where she was going to come out of this intact. He had told her so repeatedly.

'At least you have told your story now … and it's out there now,' he said. 'You should go and disappear.'

Before long, Gibson's parents started calling him at the office. Gibson, in her interview, had painted her childhood as Dickensian and burdened by unreasonable responsibilities. Natalie, Gibson's mother, wanted to tell Alex, 'Everything she said is a lie … we are great parents.'

'It was these long phone calls, with the mum on the phone and the husband yelling out the background. Soon they started asking me to put them in touch with her [Gibson]. Within about a week of the article, I just had to stop taking any of their calls.'

In the end, Gibson decided to ignore Alex's advice — that she disappear from the public eye — and, within just a few weeks, she resurfaced with an even bigger bang. Gibson had agreed to appear on *60 Minutes*, to be interviewed on camera and one-on-one with host Tara Brown. It went just as Alex had predicted.

'I think she must have been freaking out about money,' he says, 'and she must have finally cracked.' Documents that would later be filed in the Federal Court revealed that Channel Nine paid her $75,000 — through her lawyers — for the appearance on its flagship current-affairs show.

Alex had taken on Gibson as a favour for his old friend, and didn't charge for the help. But what stunned him straightaway about Gibson and her company was that there was nowhere near as much money coming in as he would have thought. He looked over their books and paid a visit to their accountants, a firm based in Fitzroy, in Melbourne's inner north. There was about $200,000 in the bank, he said, which was nothing to sneeze at. But the business appeared to be running on fumes. 'It was all mirrors.'

'They spent top-dollar on everything, a fortune on developing the app, and she got herself a nice car, nice clothes, her lease was very high,' Alex said. 'She had money coming in from the app, and an advance from Penguin, but to stay solvent they were relying on more book money coming in from sales. Meanwhile she was doing a lot of speaking gigs that were all unpaid. That's where it blew my mind. It wasn't a business to retire off. It was an average earner.

'To me, it was a shit scam. And soon as you scratched at it, it fell apart.'

THE LYING GAME

You have serious mental health issues if you conjure up lies, situations, health issues, struggles or add in [an] unreasonable amount of detail to keep things interesting … and keep up all the other lies you've told.

— Facebook post by Belle Gibson, 2014

On a warm Friday evening back in 2011, Belle Gibson walked into The Alfred hospital's neurology unit. She was 19 years old and living with her partner, her son's father, Nathan Corbett, in St Kilda East. Gibson had told doctors a few weeks earlier that she was suffering from dizziness, blurred vision, retro-orbital pain, speech problems, and breathlessness. She said she was experiencing episodes of forgetfulness, where she couldn't follow the train of conversations, or would sometimes forget her own name. Gibson reported involuntary movement, spasms of her arms and legs, and twitching of her upper lip and eye. She said her speech was sometimes slurred and that she was having problems with hand-eye coordination. She told doctors that her mother, Natalie, had MS, and that her brother, Nick, had Asperger's and epilepsy. There was a history of ischaemic heart disease, diabetes, and stroke in the family, she explained. Full blood tests and an eye examination were performed. The tests showed there was nothing wrong with Gibson; but, given they were told that her mother had been diagnosed with MS at the age of 28, she was referred for a scan anyway. At 6.19 pm on that November evening, Gibson's had a brain MRI scan, with and without a contrast.

A few weeks passed. She went back to the clinic to get the results of the scan. She had Oli with her, who was 15 months old. The consultant neurologist on duty showed her the pictures: everything was perfectly normal, he reassured her. Nothing was wrong with her brain. She did not have MS. There was no discussion whatsoever about brain cancer. If anything, the neurologist believed, Gibson was struggling with the unrelenting demands of being a new mum with little support around her. For much of their 40-minute consultation, tears streamed down Gibson's face.

After she left, the neurologist telephoned Gibson's GP. Then he followed up in writing. He told her doctor, Philip O'Reilly, from the Prahran Market Clinic, that Gibson had a 'complicated mixture' of symptoms. The visual problems and unsteadiness she reported might have been related to migraines, and the trembling and difficulty in breathing were more suggestive of panic attacks.

'Overall,' he wrote, 'I thought it highly likely from my first meeting with Annabelle that she was struggling emotionally as well as physically with her ongoing symptoms and the demands of caring for Oliver. It would appear that she has very limited assistance from family or friends. She doesn't know her father and has little contact with her mother who, of course, has her own neurological problems to contend with. Her partner Nathan does what he can to help but she could do with a lot more I feel.'

The neurologist said that Gibson 'strongly rejected' the suggestion that some of the symptoms she reported might be physical manifestations of anxiety or depression. 'She wants to know what is wrong with her and "how to fix it",' he told his colleague. The neurologist suggested some medication, and referred Gibson back to the GP. He did not believe there was any need for further investigation, but suggested that 'counselling and psychological techniques may be worthwhile'.

Gibson, by now, had been telling people for more than two years that she had a brain tumour. And a little over a year after this meeting at The Alfred hospital, where she was told by a neurologist that her MRI scan was all clear, she would log onto Instagram and claim to be beating terminal brain cancer with a healthy diet.

When Australian authorities later asked Gibson whether she had consulted any other doctors while living in Melbourne, before a second doctor cleared her of cancer, this time in 2014, her reply, through her lawyer, was that she had: 'Although Ms Gibson can't recall their names.'

Did she tell any of those GPs she had been diagnosed with cancer? If yes, who did she tell, what did she say, and when was this?

'Yes,' came the reply. 'Ms Gibson advised them of her diagnoses. Otherwise refer to above.'

The main problem with piecing together the puzzling story of Belle Gibson's health is that there are so many parts still missing. To hear her tell it, she was diagnosed with terminal brain cancer in 2009, while living in Perth. She had met a man called Mark Johns and then joined a Facebook group that he administered. A short time later, Mark, whom she believed to be an immunologist and neurologist, came over to her sharehouse, showed her some equipment, and encouraged her to join a study into the effects of the cervical cancer vaccine Gardasil.

On 25 June, Gibson was diagnosed with cancer. Mark reached this diagnosis using an 'at-home test involving his electronic diagnosis equipment'. Gibson would later claim to her followers on Facebook that Gardasil was the cause of her brain tumour. 'I got cancer from Gardasil,' she said. 'I'd prefer cervical cancer than have my time over and have the vaccination again. Gardasil poses more risks than cervical cancer itself does.' Mark showed Gibson an X-ray proving that she had brain cancer. She then called a friend (whom she no longer speaks talks to), and told him that she needed to receive treatment in Melbourne. The friend offered her a spare room in his house, and she flew over from Perth.

Gibson was expecting to meet Mark three times at the Peter MacCallum Cancer Centre. But the first meeting was cancelled. Mark, instead, drove over to her house in the suburbs of Melbourne to conduct some tests. At the second meeting, which took place in a garden near a hospital, Mark told her she was unlikely to fall pregnant. She travelled to the third appointment by tram with her then partner, Nathan, but he left to meet some friends, and Gibson waited alone. Mark never showed up, so Gibson took off. At some point, Mark had prescribed her Temodal chemotherapy medication, which she took orally. She continued to see Mark intermittently, at home, until 2011, and he would also administer radiotherapy treatment.

That is the summary of the answers that Gibson has given Australian authorities and the media when quizzed about her cancer diagnosis and treatment. But it is not the only story. When this version of events had to be massaged into something workable for Gibson's cookbook, she told it somewhat differently. This time, she claimed she was diagnosed with brain cancer around the same period, in June 2009, but then the story changes. Gibson said she received the diagnosis in a doctor's office after suffering a stroke at work. The unnamed doctor estimated that she had between six weeks and four months to live. Gibson tried chemotherapy and radiotherapy for two months, and then, one day, after vomiting and passing out in a city park opposite a hospital, she made the call to dump conventional medicine. She decided that she wasn't going to spend her last days knee-deep in nausea and other side effects of conventional treatment.

Gibson read about the detoxification properties of lemons online, and then travelled the country searching for a cure. She treated herself with nutrition and holistic medicine. 'I was empowering myself to save my own life, through nutrition, patience, determination and love,' she said, 'as well as salt, vitamin and Ayurvedic treatments, craniosacral therapy, oxygen therapy, colonics, and a whole lot of other treatments.'

But, even while Gibson was in the middle of writing the 3,000-word prologue to her book, she couldn't maintain a consistent story. In January 2014, she filled out a questionnaire asking for details of her health and medical history. On the form, she was asked to tick a box if she had ever had surgery. The box was left blank.

Do you suffer from any inherited medical conditions?
No.

Do you suffer from any current physical injuries or disabilities?
No.

Are you currently suffering any illness?
No.

Are you currently taking any prescription or non-prescription medications?
No.

**

Despite the numerous gaps in Gibson's stories, and the lack of any concrete evidence to support most of her claims, she *was* seeking alternative treatments at the time she claimed to be suffering from brain cancer. In 2014, there were rumours going around in natural-health circles about a healer by the name of Phil Best. Phil seems to exists entirely by word of mouth. He operates entirely in the shadows. He doesn't have a clinic or a website. There is no phone number listed for him online. He lives in Tasmania, but is often on the road, interstate and overseas. At one point, Phil rented a room in an alternative-health practice in Melbourne without the owners even knowing what he was qualified to do. No one seemed to check, and no one seemed to care. It didn't matter, because Phil had a reputation for getting results. People were calling him a genius.

Gibson made contact with Phil in 2014, and they met a number of times at her Elwood home, and at clinics in Melbourne and Sydney. Gibson says that Phil is the person who, in June 2014, diagnosed her with secondary cancers in her blood, spleen, uterus, and liver. According to Gibson, Phil told her that he was a doctor, and treated her with electronic equipment 'which fed data back to his computer'. Phil categorically rejects this. 'That's not true,' he said when we put this to him. 'She was diagnosed by somebody else. I didn't diagnose anything.'

Phil describes himself as a researcher and an observer, but will not say what his profession is or whether he has any qualifications in conventional or alternative medicine. He said he follows patients who are being treated in alternative-health clinics around the country, and that he's working on a book about different types of cancer treatments. Some health clinics that have been associated with Phil are vague about his role, too. One, which has since cut all ties with him, has said he promoted himself as a natural practitioner. Another saw him as a sort of go-between, who brought Gibson in for testing. Both clinics told us that they didn't pay Phil, and assumed he was being paid directly by Gibson. One person who used to work with Phil described him as an elusive character who made 'ridiculous, unfounded' claims and gave false promises. 'Some of the stuff he said he did was unbelievable, radical,' they remarked. 'A few red flags went up, so we started digging and we couldn't find anything about him.'

Phil has grey hair, and looks like he is in his 60s. He lives in a small house in the town of Devonport in northern Tasmania. When he spoke to us on the phone, he was reading the local newspaper in a library near his home while waiting for his wife to do the grocery shopping. Phil confirmed that he had met with Gibson, but denies ever diagnosing her, performing tests on her, or treating her. He says Gibson duped him; he believed her when she told him she had cancer. 'She blames everybody but herself,' Phil said. 'I didn't misrepresent the fact that she had cancer. I'm not a specialist. I just told her I was interested in research.'

But that isn't entirely true. Phil recommended that Gibson try different cancer treatments and go for expensive testing overseas. He also prescribed her a medicine cabinet full of questionable products, four days after Gibson's announced on Instagram that the cancer had metastasised. And he invoiced her for close to $9,000. Attached to the bill is a confusing, multi-coloured spreadsheet listing various treatments and their costs. Included among them are things such as a 'machine', 'capsules', and a 'travel blanket' to stop the body's 'electronic emissions and infrared radiation from dissipating outwards'. Phil told us the pills were 'enzymes and anti-inflammatory stuff'. Also listed on the invoice is a $600 charge for his monthly retainer. Gibson paid for just about everything on the bill.

Phil accompanied Gibson to GloHealth, a small clinic in Elsternwick, in Melbourne's south-east, and to Core Naturopathics, a small clinic in the suburbs of Wollongong, about an hour-and-a-half south of Sydney. One of her friends at the time, a Melbourne naturopath and health-food shop owner, flew to Sydney with her. She was concerned about Gibson going by herself. 'I was afraid,' the former friend said. 'I was worried about her travelling with brain cancer. I was worried that she was going to have a seizure.'

When the two young women landed at the airport, they were met by Phil Best. The friend remembers a scruffy-looking man wearing trousers and an ill-fitting shirt. The three of them caught the train from the airport and made their way to the clinic. On the way, Phil told them about different kinds of cancer therapies. Phil, who works in partnership with an expensive clinic in Europe, is a fervent advocate for hyperthermia, an experimental cancer treatment currently undergoing clinical trials, which involves exposing parts of the body to high temperatures.

When they arrived at the Sydney clinic, Gibson's hands and feet were connected to leads that passed a small, painless, electrical current through her body. Blood was taken from her finger and examined under a microscope. Such tests are used to build an overall picture of health and pinpoint imbalances. They cannot be used to diagnose medical conditions, but, instead, look at things like a person's fat and muscle mass, hydration levels, and blood cell structure. 'You cannot see cancer,' Core Naturopathics director, Brett O'Brien, said. Brett claimed he was told during Gibson's consultation that she had a brain tumour. He emailed Gibson her results before she posted on Instagram that her cancer had spread, but said his clinic did not give any diagnosis or advice about cancer. 'We don't make recommendations,' he said, 'and we certainly don't make recommendations about cancer.'

The friend who had travelled interstate with Gibson said it didn't take her long to reach the conclusion that Phil was not what he made himself out to be. She'd asked him about some of his treatments on the train on the way to the clinic. It didn't stack up. 'He's quite obviously a charlatan,' she said. 'He was making up all of these stories [about] treatments and testing that he did.' The former friend, backing up Gibson's version of events, said Phil was the person who diagnosed the secondary cancers. She said Gibson called her not long after their appointment and told her the news. At that point, she started to distance herself from Gibson. If she believed Phil, something was seriously wrong. 'I couldn't believe that she took something that he would say as a diagnosis,' she said. 'That's when I got as far away from her as possible. At that point, I still believed that she had a brain tumour, but when she rung me and said that Phil gave her that diagnosis I thought, *I am staying away from you*. I thought, *Y-o-u-r-e … c-r-a-z-y*.'

Importantly, it is worth noting here that months earlier, back in March 2014, Gibson had been telling her publisher that she was being tested for secondary cancer. 'Cell abnormalities have come back, but still inconclusive,' she told Penguin. Then, a couple of weeks later, she sent a text message to a friend who was checking in with her after a supposed doctor's appointment, saying: 'Sample came back malignant. Got more bloods taken. Going back in for ultrasound Monday x.'

In a text message to another friend, just after 7.15 pm on 17 March 2014, Gibson said, 'I'm really sick.'

Friend: Talk to me … You got your test results back? Xx

Gibson: Yep. They found more.

Friend: More cancer? Where?

Gibson: Yep. I can't breathe. I'm so sad. Spleen and liver.

But there was no doctor's appointment and no test results. The last time Gibson had seen a doctor was three years earlier, when a brain scan showed that she was perfectly healthy. Months before she even met Phil Best, Gibson was talking about secondary cancers. And six months after meeting him, when Gibson finally went to a GP for tests and was told definitively that she did not have cancer, she kept on pretending she did. Later, she claimed she didn't tell Apple because she did not update the company 'on health or personal matters'; asked why she didn't inform Penguin, her lawyer submitted that she 'was in shock and denial' after having been cleared of cancer. 'Ms Gibson has been working with a psychologist to understand this time,' the lawyer said.

Whatever the explanation, what is clear is that Gibson was still spinning stories right up until the very end. In March 2015, as the news articles piled up and everything was unravelling around her, she continued telling the people closest to her about fake medical dramas. This time, she claimed, she was about to undergo surgery.

Allison was dying. She was 35 years old, single, and working as a corporate secretary when she was diagnosed with breast cancer. It was the rapidly progressive type; the type that had already metastasised. And it was going to kill her. When Allison told her co-workers about the prognosis, there was an immediate outpouring of sympathy and warmth. She was embraced, too, by the women she met in a breast-cancer support group at the local Duke University campus, near her home in Durham, North Carolina. Allison had always struggled to make friends, but at these meetings had no difficulty striking friendships easily. All who went there had something terrible in common. Week after week, over the course of two years, as Allison shed her hair and lost more than 25 kilograms, those bonds grew stronger.

Marc Feldman, an American psychiatrist, had just started a new job in 1989 at Duke University Medical Center when he received a telephone call. It was from the chairman of the psychiatry department. He wanted Marc to take on a new case. Marc was one of the newest members of the faculty, so he felt he didn't have much choice in the matter. It was the policy that newcomers like him accepted every case referred their way by the more senior colleagues. 'And I'm glad that was the policy,' says Marc, from his home office in Alabama, 'because this one patient set me on my career path.' The patient referred to Marc for evaluation was Allison. She'd voluntarily admitted herself into hospital. She was distraught.

Marc met her in one of the psychiatry wards at Duke University Hospital. She told him she had overwhelming anxiety and dysphoria. 'I've been acting like a compulsive liar,' Allison said in their first meeting. The leaders of Allison's cancer support group had grown concerned, suspecting she wasn't telling the truth about her illness. They had done some digging, and discovered she had never met the oncologist who she claimed was treating her. They confronted her. Allison started off denying it, but eventually came clean. It was all a ruse. She was not, as she had claimed, dying from cancer. She wasn't physically sick. The next day, she told her boss, and was fired.

Marc learnt that the story had begun a couple of years earlier when Allison was left broken-hearted after her fiancé met someone else and ended their engagement. She felt betrayed and abandoned. Then, one day, she woke up, went into work, and told everyone she was dying from cancer. Allison even copied the appearance of an acquaintance who had breast cancer: she shaved her head to look like a chemotherapy patient, started wearing a wig, and dieted to lose an extreme amount of weight. Allison didn't want to appear 'too well', so she started turning down invitations to social events. Once, suspecting that people become too complacent about her terminal prognosis, she invented a story about her grandfather being severely injured in a fire.

Marc initially thought that Allison was malingering. But malingerers, he points out, are people who feign sickness for a specific reason, such as to get out of work or to gain financial compensation. Allison's motives were less tangible. She wanted to be nurtured; she wanted sympathy. Her illness was more fitting with a factitious disorder. In the Diagnostic and Statistical Manual of Mental Disorders (DSM-5), factitious disorder is characterised as faking symptoms of illness, or inducing injury or disease, 'even in the absence of obvious external rewards'. Onset is often in early adulthood after a legitimate hospitalisation for a physical or mental condition. One of the most severe factitious disorders is Munchausen Syndrome, where a person fakes or induces illness to get attention or sympathy. The disorder is named after Baron von Münchhausen, an eighteenth-century German officer who had a reputation for embellishing stories about his military adventures. His name was later appropriated for the title of a book by German writer Rudolf Erich Raspe, which was published in 1785.

In the late 1980s, Marc hadn't heard of this syndrome, or, for that matter, any case of medical deception. During years of study at Dartmouth Medical School and then residency training, where he treated hundreds of patients, the idea that someone would fake being sick simply had never come up. Indeed, Munchausen syndrome was a relatively new condition, having first made an appearance in medical literature in 1951.

Marc was intrigued. He decided to write up Allison's case for a medical journal, and in the spring of 1991 it was published under the headline, 'The Longing for Nurturance: a case of factitious cancer.' He explained that, during her treatment, Allison was forthcoming and remorseful. She seemed relieved that it was all over, that she could stop pretending, that she could stop living a lie. Marc diagnosed her with major depression and mixed personality disorder.

He prescribed antidepressants, and she continued her therapy. After a month in hospital, she was discharged and moved interstate to start a new life. In the article, Marc wrote that for some people, 'loneliness and isolation may lead them well beyond direct requests for support, even to the intricate enactment of a terminal illness'. The article caught the attention of local media, and *The Los Angeles Times* ran a story about the condition.

Immediately, Marc was barraged with new reported cases. People were seeking him out for an opinion on this little-known condition that, much like a physical disease, infects everyone the patient comes into contact with. Marc, who found the subject utterly fascinating, embraced his new role and, in the subsequent three decades, became an authority in the field. Through his website, hundreds of people from around the world contact him every year asking for advice. Now a clinical professor of psychiatry at the University of Alabama, he is regularly summoned as an expert witness in court cases, usually for the defence in personal injury and malpractice claims, where there's an allegation of medical deception. He's also working on his fourth book about factitious disorders, Munchausen Syndrome, and Munchausen by proxy, where a person — often a mother — makes their child sick to get attention.

A few years ago, Marc noticed that something new was starting to happen. Just like in real life, people were feigning illness online. They joined forums and chat rooms and started blogs, and they pretended to have everything from leukaemia to anorexia to paraplegia. Marc coined the term *Munchausen by Internet* (which is not currently a recognised form of the disorder in the DSM-5). As with Munchausen, these people identify as a patient, a fighter, or a survivor, and they crave attention, sympathy, and control.

Marc has never met or assessed Belle Gibson. At face value, there appears to be similarities between her online behaviour and what Marc and others have described. But without a clinical assessment, it is impossible to diagnose a person with any condition. She has a long history of making up grandiose stories, which she may, in part, believe. And she has acknowledged that she has a problem telling the truth. This *could* point to a mental illness. But without Gibson's medical records, we may never know what motivated her to act in the way she did.

One of the biggest questions people have about Munchausen syndrome is whether the person claiming to be ill knows that what they are doing is wrong. The answer, Marc says, is yes. They know they are lying. This is evident because of the elaborate planning that goes into carrying out the deception. What they don't always understand is *why*; what drives them to lie in the first place. But the answer to that question is far more complicated.

Marc says that many of these patients share a few things in common. First, they have experienced emotional abuse or neglect in childhood. Second, they have received medical treatment for a real, serious ailment during childhood; it's likely that this is where they learned that manufacturing illness is the only guaranteed way to get the attention and nurturance they crave. The third common thread among this cohort of patients is a personality disorder, such as borderline personality disorder, which usually begin to manifest in adolescence. As the DSM-5 says, a factitious disorder would only be diagnosed if a person's behaviour was not better explained by another mental disorder, such as a delusional disorder or a psychotic disorder.

The sad catch-22 scenario for people with Munchausen syndrome is that they are viewed by those who know them as manipulative. And after a while, friends and family report feeling victimised, and start to avoid them. But this can fuel the person's feelings of isolation and, in turn, increase the appeal of being deceptive.

Marc says these patients generally resist psychiatric treatment, and when they do attend, they don't respond well. He likens people with Munchausen syndrome to travelling performers, moving from town to town, city, or even country once they're exposed, to start all over again, sending medical staff on wild goose chases for conditions that simply don't exist.

18

NO MONEY, NO HONEY

One afternoon, a couple of weeks after the *Australian Women's Weekly* ran its interview with Gibson in which she admitted her cancer was a lie, the phone rang at Bauer Media Group's head office on Park Street in Sydney. The agitated person on the end of the line demanded to speak with Ita Buttrose, the crusading editor of the magazine who was appointed by the late Kerry Packer in the mid-1970s. The call was put through to Bryce Corbett. He explained that Ita had long since left the company, formerly Australian Consolidated Press, founded by the patriarch of the Packer family, Sir Frank, in the 1930s.

Somewhere in the midst of that long conversation, the person on the other end of the line identified herself as *her* mother. Bryce didn't know what she meant.

'*Belle Gibson's*,' the woman finally said.

Bryce kept asking questions. Eventually, he realised it was possible that he was actually talking to Gibson's mother, Natalie, and to her husband, Andrew Dal Bello. 'It was just rambling,' Corbett recalls. 'They were all about, "We're going to sue you because you brought our family name into disrepute."'

Bryce, an experienced newspaper and magazine journalist, smelled a story. May's edition of the magazine with Gibson had generated lots of press coverage and publicity, and had sold very well. Securing an exclusive with her mother the following month would be yet another coup. He offered them a platform to tell *their* side of the story.

'Suddenly, the conversation went from me being the worst person in the world to, "Oh, darling, Oh, I don't know, sweetheart, Oh, what would I wear? We've got so much on."

'And so the dance began.'

The deadline for the magazine's next issue was fast approaching, but if Bryce could get the Dal Bellos from their home in Adelaide, South Australia, to Sydney within 24 hours, there was an outside chance he could hold the printers and get the story on the page in time.

After a few more phone calls and the promise of accommodation and return flights via Brisbane to visit their son, Nick, the Dal Bellos agreed to get on the last plane out of Adelaide that day. The magazine sent a taxi to pick them up from their home and ferry them to the airport. The cab waited outside their house for 40 minutes; by the time they finally arrived at the airport, the gate was closed. There were tears at the check-in desk, Bryce recalls.

'I remember having a long phone call with the poor girl on the Virgin desk in Adelaide Airport, and Natalie's in the background just wailing because they missed the plane, and it was all a disaster and nobody understands, and Andrew was there trying to placate her. This poor Virgin employee was saying, "I don't know what to do with them." I said to her, "Can you just look after them, just keep them in your sight for 20 minutes while I work out what I'm going to do?"'

Bryce managed to get the Dal Bellos into a room in a nearby airport motel, and re-booked them on a flight the following day. He laughs at the recollection of receiving the motel bill after they checked out. 'They just went to town,' he says. 'Ordered everything on the menu — everything out of the mini bar they could get their hands on. The bill was about as outrageous as you can get for a restaurant in an airport motel!'

Waiting for them to arrive in Sydney, Bryce fully expected the Dal Bellos to pack up, turn around, and head home. But they didn't. Natalie and Andrew touched down, where Bryce and journalist Clair Weaver were waiting. The four of them went out for dinner at the Opera Bar at the Sydney Opera House, overlooking the Sydney Harbour Bridge.

It was a surreal experience, according to Bryce. 'Clair and I spent most the night trying to make sense of the madness,' he says. 'Natalie seemed to veer from being vaguely threatening to being our long-lost aunt. She would occasionally slur her words, and talked a lot about various illnesses that meant she had to take a series of meds. By the end of the night, we seemed to have inadvertently become part of the family. "You must come to Adelaide," both Natalie and Andrew insisted. "Come and stay with us. It would be wonderful, darling."'

After dinner overlooking the harbour, the Dal Bellos checked into their hotel, the Ibis Sydney World Square, on Pitt Street in the central business district. The next day, they were picked up and taken down to the magazine's studio in Alexandria for make-up, styling, and the mandatory magazine photoshoot. Bryce says he and Clair interviewed the couple throughout, and the more they heard, the more difficult it became to know what was true and what wasn't. Bryce had asked Natalie to bring a box of documents with her — birth certificates, school reports, drivers' licences — anything that would help to establish both her identity and that of her daughter. As the photographer went about her work, Bryce and Clair pored over the documentary evidence. There was no doubt she was Belle Gibson's mother. And, indeed, if there were any doubt at all, it was extinguished the minute the photos started appearing on the screen. The family likeness was remarkable. Both journalists came away from the encounter with the impression that the tangled web that was Gibson's family life went a long way to explaining her apparent confusion.

'You kind of went, "Woooaaahhh …"' Bryce says.

The interview in the *Weekly* was the first of two that the Dal Bellos gave. In it, Natalie spoke out against her estranged daughter, disputing details of her upbringing, and criticising her for 'playing the victim card'. It was a public and brutal attack. Natalie told the national magazine's 1.6 million readers that she doubted her daughter was 'capable of empathy'.

'I can't tell you how embarrassed we are about what she has done,' Natalie said. 'And we sincerely wish to apologise to anyone who was deceived by Belle. For what small part we played in her life, we would like to say sorry.'

Then, in a second interview, two months later, with Melbourne's *Herald Sun*, Natalie called for her daughter to be left alone, and described Gibson's con as a 'white lie'.

'Belle is allowed to tell little porky pies,' she told the paper. 'Who the hell doesn't tell a lie in their life? Nobody complained about Belle when she was helping people and now they want to put her under the microscope.'

It was clear that Gibson's relationship with her mother and stepfather was fractured, but it was also apparent there was much more to this family's complicated story.

The initial meeting with the couple, and the months-long

hangover from it, was something that Bryce and Clair had never before experienced. For months after the story came out, they received daily phone calls from the Dal Bellos. There seemed to be an emotional neediness behind this. Eventually, they just had to stop answering.

Bryce summed it bluntly: 'Each time you answered the phone, it was like opening the front door on a tornado. You'd hear the voice and know you were in for a good half-hour of stream of consciousness. And the more you heard, the more you learned, the more you started to wonder about the kind of childhood Belle had had.'

The radio is playing loudly in the background of the recorded voicemail message. It's halfway through Kylie Minogue's 2001 dance song, *Can't Get You Out of My Head*. The woman has a thick Australian accent, and speaks slowly. Her voice is breathy. It stretches and stammers down the phone line.

The 28-second recording goes like this:

> *La la la* … Sorry we're busy at the moment, can you please leave a brief message, or a text, after the tone … *I just can't get you out of my head* … much appreciated, have a nice day … *Boy, your lovin' is all I think about* … and, um, take care and be careful … and the best time to contact us would be lunchtime onwards. Thank you. Due to circumstances … *Every night, every day* … Bye.

When Natalie Dal Bello answers the phone, on a Tuesday afternoon, she's straight away suspicious, paranoid even. Only three people have her phone number, and she wants to know where we got it from. We tell her, but she doesn't believe us. Then she drops that line of questioning and asks how she can help.

A phone call with Belle Gibson's mother has its own peculiar rhythm. She listens to questions, but doesn't always answer them. And she asks the same questions more than once. She forgets things, and seems to struggle to hang on to her thoughts. Sometimes, she gets muddled and can't find the right words. Sometimes, she slurs. At times, she is incoherent. The conversations are always long. So are goodbyes.

During the first call, Natalie discusses her medical conditions and those of other family members. She's glowing about Gibson's education, employment history, her looks, and her upbringing. She blasts phony doctors — the ones who she says tricked her daughter, the one who removed her husband's appendix, and the one who nearly killed her by prescribing 42 pills a day. The conversation chops and changes; it covers the media, and the weather in different capital cities. Natalie says she doesn't use the computer or go on the internet. She keeps up to date with Gibson's court case through local Adelaide radio station Mix 102.3FM.

Natalie is a thickset woman in her mid-50s. She has dark hair, wears red lipstick, and walks with a cane. In the *Weekly's* photoshoot, she wears two sets of gold hoop earrings. A gold necklace with a charm of St Christopher, the patron saint of travellers, hangs around her neck. The similarities between her and Gibson are striking: they have the same wide grin and dimples. Natalie is a proud woman. She is proud of her kids — she says she has six, although her own mother says there are only five — and of her grandkids. Natalie adores her 'wonderful husband', Andrew, whom she lovingly refers to as her 'country man'.

Andrew, in his late 50s, is from a big Italian family. He was a welder for 41 years, earning $17 an hour, he says, before being struck down by illness. He has short brown hair and wears large, rectangular, black-rimmed glasses. Most calls with Natalie are within earshot of Andrew, who seems to be always pottering around in the background.

Natalie and Andrew refuse all our requests for a sit-down interview in their home, and they won't tell us where they live. 'Not even some of our family knows,' says Andrew. For some reason, they want us to believe they live in the country. But that's not true. They used to rent a brick house in a working-class northern suburb of Adelaide, but moved after they got married in 2012. Natalie says before that they lived in Brisbane, but moved interstate after the 2011 floods. When the *Australian Women's Weekly* sent a taxi to their house, it picked them up from an address in the same Adelaide neighbourhood where Andrew last rented a house. Bryce Corbett remembers it being public housing.

Sometimes, the Dal Bellos open up; sometimes, they're cagey. During the first phone call, Natalie seems uninhibited and happy. Andrew is less forthcoming. He seizes the phone, and his gruff voice pipes down the line. It's an avalanche of words. There is no introduction. Andrew says they won't be giving interviews without being paid.

'If you want to do an interview, we're happy to do an interview, but we won't actually do it for charity, OK? What are you happy to put on the table? I'm telling you that we don't work for charity, OK?'

'I do,' Natalie says, in the background.

'Yeah, you do.'

'I do it out of my own pocket,' she says, taking the phone back.

'They can call us back some other time,' Andrew can be heard saying, as he disappears.

Natalie starts talking.

'I've got a very good background,' she says. 'I've worked, my husband and myself, and all the family members are working very, very hard, we've paid a lot of taxes through our life, I do a lot of charity work free of charge, and none of our family members have a criminal record, and, you know, that's all I can really say at the moment.'

But she goes on without a pause. Her words come out in a twisted knot.

Natalie says the media spotlight on her family has been devastating. 'Absolutely devastating,' she says. 'Enough to say that it's caused me to be terminal, and my husband is terminal, with our health. It is actually devastating, and I don't understand because we've given Annabelle everything she wanted, we financed her lifestyle to a certain point, OK?

'As I said, I'm married to a country man, I've got beautiful children, and as I said, we are all well educated, never been neglected, OK, and Annabelle did have everything she wanted, OK, so I don't understand. I think it's the taste in life, this social media especially, the addiction, the addiction now with young men and women is that when they've got too much of a champagne lifestyle they want more and more and more as they get older.'

'They can't stop themselves,' Andrew chimes in.

'OK?' says Natalie. 'Where I had my champagne lifestyle when I was younger. So now I, sort of, I don't wear make-up, you know, 24 hours a day, and, you know, a few hundred rings or necklaces or what have you.'

Natalie and Andrew say they are a close-knit and hard-working family. They want to be seen as good, charitable, salt-of-the-earth people. Natalie says she studied beauty therapy, and talks a lot about her volunteer work, which, she says, includes mentoring newly arrived refugees and caring for six non-English-speaking Saudi Arabian children for up to 14 hours a day in her home, free of charge. As with most things the Dal Bellos claim, there is no way to verify this.

In the first call, Gibson's older brother, Nick, who is visiting his mother from Brisbane, where he lives with his son, comes on to the phone. His words come out in rapid fire. He doesn't listen until he's finished making his point.

'I know my sister might have done a lot of mistakes, but we all make mistakes, mate, alright? Believe me, I've made a lot of mistakes as well. I'm a dad to a five-year-old. He's not a mistake, but I've done a lot of other mistakes in my time. But, you know, what people are saying about my baby sister, it's just not right, it's hurtful, and yeah, maybe my baby sister might have said a lot of things about me on media, it might be a load of crap, but at the end of the day she was trying to get attention. It's not very fair. You know, not on her and not on my family. And what newspaper are you guys from?'

Nick says he's been estranged from Gibson, but wants her back in his life. They have sons about the same age. There is nothing he would love more than to see his little sister.

'I don't hate my sister for what she's done to me or my family, for what she's said. You know, I messaged her a few weeks ago to wish her a happy birthday, and I got a reply back. Before those messages came through I wasn't talking to my sister for a long, long time, you know, so I was quite happy to even get that one message. I got one reply back saying, "Thanks", and that's it, but that message is enough for me to have a smile on my face.

'My sister's not a bad person. She's a mother, she's a parent to a little boy. At the end of the day, we've all got medical problems. If my sister didn't have cancer, it's something else she's got wrong with her. I've got a bad shoulder, I've got a bad knee from football, you know, we've all got a medical problem, but most of the time we can't see that medical problem.'

Over the course of half-a-dozen phone calls to the Dal Bello household, it becomes clear that they keep odd hours; the phone always rings out in the mornings.

Natalie and Andrew are storytellers. They like to chat. The conversations switch abruptly from the intimate details of their lives, to the mundane, to the seemingly unbelievable. They talk about being forced to move house after a home invasion, and about a murder plot they claim was aimed at them. They continue to say they are private people, practically housebound, but then they open up to journalists, strangers whom they have never met, disclosing the most personal kind of information. During hours and hours of phone calls, Natalie and Andrew bounce off each other, and they interrupt each other, regularly passing their old prepaid Nokia mobile back and forth to interject.

Natalie says her daughter is a smart woman — not a liar nor calculating — and claims that she definitely was not neglected as a child.

'She could go anywhere in life, and I mean anywhere,' Natalie explains. 'I'm not saying that she's a person who's going to give a hell of a lot in life without her coming, probably first, to a certain degree, but I am definitely saying that she's done some pretty special things in life as well, and she's very gifted. And as you see, she's got her beauty. If she stays off social media she can probably get her life back on track.'

Both Natalie and Andrew think very little of Clive, Gibson's partner. Natalie says her daughter can do better, and they agree that Clive is the mastermind behind The Whole Pantry, despite there being no evidence of this. Natalie says Gibson genuinely believed she had cancer and that she was hospitalised in Perth with a leaking valve in her heart. Later, she says her daughter has heart disease, but is unable to provide any other consistent information about her medical history. Sometimes, she says Gibson has 'done no wrong' and has been manipulated by others.

Then she blasts the media.

'If I knew that I had one day to live, believe me, word for word, and you can print this if you want, I'd get someone from Melbourne, probably from the Italian or Greek mafia, and, believe me, I would definitely make sure that people in media, and that's not you, Beau, that they'd be paying for it. You remember, Annabelle's the baby of the family, and she's very articulated, and despite whether anyone wants to think we've done something wrong, which we haven't, OK, or she didn't get her favourite teddy bear, would you believe that we would even go as far as Toowoomba, OK, if she lost a teddy bear or something? We'd go back to the same florist or baby shop just to get the same teddy bear, OK, to make sure that she'd have the same thing that she may have lost.'

One time, Natalie says she can't feel her fingers, and passes the phone to Andrew. He comes on to the line, and starts ranting about social-media addiction, how it's the same as heroin addiction. He talks fast and loudly, and is uninterruptible. Then he gets to Gibson's book.

'Put it this way,' he says. 'It wouldn't do you any harm even if you was frickin' dying, it would still help you, OK. There's nothing in that book that she says that you would take that would actually kill you. The only thing that she actually fucked up on is the cancer bit — if she left that out it'd be a perfect book, OK, it's as simple as that. And the cancer thing was to sell the fucken book, because people fucken got cancer fucken every day, there's that many people diagnosed, there's an open market there.'

Natalie takes the phone back.

'The book was great until things unfolded,' she says. 'And would you believe she's the most remarkable cook you could imagine?'

Later, when Andrew criticises the book, Natalie fires back at him: 'Excuse me, but her book could still cure cancer,' she tells him.

You get the feeling the Dal Bellos haven't actually read the book.

Over the hours, Natalie and Andrew detail their own medical conditions. Natalie lists multiple sclerosis, breathing difficulties, a heart condition, leaky veins, a fractured knee, and more among the ailments afflicting her. She says she has spores on her lungs after living through the two Brisbane floods. One time, she says she survived cancer in 1982. At another point, she says she has cancer. Later, again, she says she's on borrowed time and has been given only months to live. Andrew, they tell us, is suffering from depression, has a spinal-cord problem, and is dying from emphysema.

Sometimes, during the calls, Natalie volunteers permission to record the audio. Other times, sometimes minutes later, she warns against taping her. Sometimes, Andrew talks about hiring a lawyer, and threatens to sue — us and Penguin — for pain and suffering. Natalie asks what the story will be and in which newspaper it will appear. She asks if we work with Bryce or Clair from the *Weekly*, or Rebecca Cavanagh, a *Herald Sun* journalist. We tell her no, and she seems suspicious, but always keeps talking.

Natalie can be forward and flirtatious. 'I'm going to smack your backside,' she once says, giggling. Another time, when she answers the phone, she asks if it's a 'booty call'. After the third phone call, she sent a picture message with a professional-looking headshot. In it, her brunette hair is long and styled, falling over rounded shoulders. The frame cuts off above her strapless top. She wears bright-red lipstick and a half smile, her head is tilted, and her gaze is back towards the camera. 'Ur mrs love u heaps. Miss u darling xoxo,' the accompanying text read.

Natalie has a high-pitched, raspy laugh that sounds as if it rises up from the belly. You imagine her throwing her head back when she finds something funny, and then turning to Andrew to repeat the joke or an amusing piece of new information. Sometimes, Natalie pulls away from the phone to relay something to her husband. If Andrew is in another room, or outside, she shouts out to him. He always shouts back.

Natalie always asks about her daughter. They're estranged, but she won't say why, or how long it's been since they last spoke. She knows very little about Gibson's life — where she lives, who she lives with. Natalie wants us to send recent photos of her, the Northcote house, Clive. She asks many questions about her daughter. Has she been posting online? Is she still in a relationship with Clive? How much older is he? Is he behind the whole thing? When is her next court date? Why does she not have a lawyer? Will we tell her to get a lawyer? Why is the media out to get her? What has she done that is so wrong?

They ask us to send information about Gibson's court case, but won't give their address. They want it delivered to their local post office at Clearview Plaza, an inner-city suburb of Adelaide.

After a few more calls, Natalie and Andrew are on the same page: they both want money for an interview in person. Failing that, Natalie wants to be flown to Melbourne for a holiday. Or to Brisbane to meet Nick's new daughter, her new grandchild. There's a bigger story here anyway, explains Andrew: his life story, which he plans to pen and sell to a Hollywood producer, 'before I die in about 10 years'.

'I'll tell you one thing,' Andrew says, his voice piping down the phone line. 'Nothing in this world is for nothing, OK? I've worked hard, my Natalie's worked very hard, OK? We do a lot of work for charity and people that we do help, so we would want something to pass on to our charities for our effort, OK?'

We always say no. But the Dal Bellos alway volunteer more information, and they always steer the conversation back to money. Sometimes, at the end of a call, Natalie doesn't hang up the phone.

The Dal Bellos can be heard talking about how much they could get from selling their story to us. Two thousand dollars is the least they will take. They also talk about selling Gibson's grandmother's phone number and home address to the media for 'top dollar'. And Natalie cautions her husband about being gruff on the phone: 'Believe me, you get more with a honey pot then you do with vinegar,' she tells him.

During one of our last phone calls, Natalie is talking about the different places Gibson lived as a child. Then she stops. 'You're good at fishing, baby,' she says. 'Darling, I think you want a free story. If Fairfax gives me money, believe me I'll have a party with homeless people. Darling, it's a multibillion-dollar company, for God's sake.'

'Tell him no money, no honey,' Andrew shouts in the background.

'No money, no honey,' Natalie repeats, slurring.

'That's the way the world works,' Andrew says, disappearing again.

'Would you believe that I would give the world to anybody?' asks Natalie. 'And if you hang up, that's OK, but I trust you, OK? And to trust me and earn my trust, believe me, that's pretty special. I think you should talk to the accounting department because, believe me, I want to see you go places as well. If you read the *Womens Weekly*, that was just a taste. I've got lots to tell you.'

19

PUBLIC SHAMING

'Good evening,' intoned host Tara Brown, opening Sunday night's *60 Minutes* program on 28 June 2015. 'A young, beautiful woman gets given the terrible news she had inoperable brain cancer and only four months to live. The courageous Belle Gibson tries chemotherapy and radiotherapy, but no luck, so turns to alternative medicine to battle the disease … it seems to work, as she tells the world through social media. Hundreds of thousands of sympathetic followers and fellow sufferers live every step of her journey and celebrate her success as she becomes the poster girl for the alternative wellness industry.

'There's an award-winning app and a cookbook. Belle Gibson has made it. Except it's all a lie. A great big lie.'

The camera flashed to Gibson. She was waiting beneath the light in the darkened room where the program's producers had set everything up. The crew were all out of the frame now, but they were standing all around her. Gibson was wearing a bright-pink turtleneck jumper, and had her hair pulled back in a ponytail. She was sitting very still.

'Will she finally tell the truth?'

Gibson was not a complete novice. She had been in front of the camera many times before. She had been filmed and photographed, and had made speeches at the podiums of star-studded award ceremonies. In 2013, she was interviewed live on Australia's most-watched breakfast TV show, *Sunrise*, where she was introduced as a mother and businesswoman who was living with brain cancer. She exhibited poise and good posture; she exuded grace and confidence. She beamed, and shared laughs with her hosts, who looked on at her in awe and asked her questions like, 'For a person living with brain cancer — and might I add you look incredibly healthy — what are your top tips for health?'.

But that was then, and this was now. Her appearance on *60 Minutes* would be nothing like that. When you've committed the sort of sins that Gibson had, and your explanation doesn't stack up, no amount of media exposure can prepare you for the hard-nosed hammering of veteran interviewers like Tara Brown. Their questions will make your toes curl. They will not relent, or wave through inexactitudes. And by dissecting one fact at a time, they will splinter your credibility.

Four months had passed since *The Age*'s first revelations about Gibson were published. She had since confessed to the *Australian Women's Weekly* that she did not have cancer, although she had stopped short of saying she was sorry for lying. Tonight's *60 Minutes* was going to be one of two things: either her chance to explain and to apologise and to make sense of behaviour that has been so widely slammed as so utterly reprehensible; or she would be torn to shreds, in perhaps the most public of bloodlettings. Either way, with more than 1.07 million viewers tuned in to watch, this was the most important interview of Gibson's life.

Tara opened her inquisition by unpicking the biggest mistruth of all the mistruths in Gibson's tangled story. She began with the introductory pages of her book, *The Whole Pantry*:

> I will never forget sitting alone in the doctor's office three weeks later waiting for my test results. He called me in and said, 'You have malignant brain cancer, Belle. You're dying. You have six weeks, four months tops'.

'But there was no real doctor,' a voiceover said, 'no doctor's office, and no conventional test results, as most people would expect and demand. It's highly questionable, but this is Belle's revised story now. She says in 2009 she met a man called Mark Johns, who told her he was an immunologist and neurologist, though no record of him exists.'

The screen returned to the interview room. 'He had come to my home and went through a series of tests,' Gibson said.

'So he comes to your home and does some tests on you?'

'Mm. He does.'

'What sort of tests?,' Tara inquired.

'It was a box, a machine, with lights on the front and that was apparently German technology. There's a — two pads, two metal pads, one that goes below the chair and one that goes behind your back, and then that measures what I believe, or remember to be, frequencies.'

'And what were the results?'

Gibson stopped. She exhaled. She looked down at her lap. She paused for eight seconds, but it felt like even longer. 'He said to me that I had a stage-four brain tumour … and that I had approximately four months to live.'

'Why,' Tara instantly continued, 'did you write in the foreword of your book that you got this information in your doctor's office, that you got this prognosis in your doctor's office?'

'Because I think that being open and telling people the way it happened would not be understood —'

'So you were —'

'— and that people would be disappointed or angry for me, you know, not following what is the right way to go about this.'

'So you lied because you feared you wouldn't be believed?' Tara asked. 'Is that what you're saying?'

'It's not what I'm saying.'

'Well, can you be clearer on what you're saying? I mean, you were absolutely misleading, weren't you? You said a doctor gave you this terrible prognosis in his office, and you've just admitted that you didn't say it was at your home and it wasn't with a real doctor because you thought people would be disappointed in you.'

'I believed he was real. No. I believed he was a real doctor.'

'So, did you lie to be believed, is the question?'

'I didn't see him in his doctor's office in Perth.'

'You didn't see him in his doctor's office ever, because he doesn't have an office, does he?'

'No.'

'Right. You also claimed in your book that you underwent chemotherapy and radiotherapy for two months.'

'Yeah.'

'True or false?'

'At the time —'

'True or false?'

'True. Because at the time, I believed I was having radiotherapy.'

'So, false?'

'I believed that I was having radiotherapy.'

Gibson looked uneasy. Her voice quivered, and her eyes darted, and she often hesitated for far too long. She repeatedly evaded yes-

or-no questions by launching into long stories.

'It just seems like you chose to believe you had cancer,' Tara said.

'Nobody wants to live with the fear of a terminal illness or dying.'

'No, and nobody knows that better than people who actually live with that, and you didn't live with that — that's not what you had.'

'No, it's not, but I lived for years with the fear that I was dying, and that is horrible, and I'm still coming to terms with that — I can take that off my shoulders now.'

'Did you live in fear of being found out?'

'No. Because I wasn't living in a space where I didn't know that this wasn't my reality.'

'Would you accept that you're a pathological liar?'

'No.'

Tara kept pointing out all of the inconsistencies that were making her claims so implausible. She implored her to just *tell the truth*. But Gibson was unable to give a straight answer on even the most basic facts.

'OK, Belle,' Tara said, cutting her off, 'this is a really, really simple question. How old are you?'

'I believe I'm 26. I have two — two birth certificates, and I've had my name changed four times. The identity crisis there is big, but that was my normal when I was growing up, Tara.'

'What do you know the truth to be now?'

'That's probably a question that we'll have to keep digging for, because it's not something I've ever understood or had answers around.'

'So, when you needed to file some financial documents, how did you choose the birthdate you gave?'

'With my most recent deed-poll paper, which has the younger of the age and the most recent of the name.'

'Right, so, currently then, according to these documents, you're 23.'

'Correct.'

Printed across Gibson's headshot on the Learner's Permit she got after moving to Melbourne was her birthdate, showing she was 23.

At one point, Tara just closed her eyes, started shaking her head, and put one hand up to stop Gibson mid-sentence. 'Belle, Belle, *Belle*, Belle, *please*,' she said. 'I mean, either you are interested in getting to the bottom of this and presenting the facts as they are — the facts — or you are not.' Gibson was stammering. Her claims were conflicting and outlandish. But she kept returning to her core message: she had actually believed she was sick at the time, and did not knowingly deceive. *I've not been intentionally untruthful.*

Tara would later describe how frustrating it was to be 'on the other end of her lies'. It was clear there would be no proper remorse on Gibson's part for her actions, or an admission of guilt. So the interview became a demolition job, a modern-day public lashing. Tara cast back even further: to Gibson's habit over many years of making up stories of suffering astonishing medical conditions in an apparent bid to 'gain maximum sympathy'. Her lies are still enshrined today in old chat forums on the internet.

'So, 2009 was a really bad year for you, wasn't it? You had three heart operations, suffered two cardiac arrests, died twice on the operating table, you had a stroke, and you were diagnosed with an inoperable brain tumour and given four months to live.'

'Correct,' Gibson replied. 'And I do ... I still have the heart condition, and I was supposed to have surgery for that.'

'You were supposed to have surgery ...'

'And I didn't.'

'Why did you tell people you had three surgeries?'

'At the time, I think, going back, I was late teens, and I was going through a lot of emotional trauma and a lot of abuse at the time.'

'What sort of abuse?'

'Um, someone who was really prominent during my childhood was, ah, stalking me.'

At the time in question, the voiceover said, Gibson was living in Perth and was a frequent contributor to an online skateboarding forum. 'But instead of chatting about skateboarding, Belle was telling her friends an elaborate fairy tale, supposedly from her hospital bed, in not one but three admissions for life-saving heart surgery.'

'Were you in hospital at the times you were posting these?' said Tara, her eyebrows raised.

'No.'

'You go into extraordinary details ... *I had surgery about seven hours ago ... the doctor comes in and tells me the draining failed and I went into cardiac arrest and died for just under three minutes. I had the most intense bruising from the paddles when they electrocuted me back to consciousness.*'

'See, I haven't read back through all of that,' Gibson said. 'But I also think that when you are young and have gone through the situation I had just gone through, you are melodramatic.'

'Melodramatic?' Tara scoffed. 'They are straight-out lies! You weren't in hospital, and you were claiming you were. Claimed you'd died twice; you didn't. Claimed you had two cardiac arrests; you didn't. That's not melodramatic. That's straight-out lying — extraordinary lies. If you lie about that, and you go to those extraordinary lengths to create the story around that lie, how can we believe anything you say now?'

'Tara, I have lost everything. And I'm not here to regain it. But when you hit rock bottom there is only an opportunity to be honest and to heal and to apologise. And I'm here to do that. There is no reason for me to lie, and it's not something I want to be doing either.'

It didn't really matter what she was saying anymore — whether she believed she had lied or not. Gibson was right about one thing:

her stocks *were* at rock bottom. #BelleGibson was trending on Twitter, and the verdict was unanimous. No one believed a word she was saying:

This Belle Gibson bird is an absolute fucking moron

LIAR. YOU ARE LYING!

She is a compulsive liar — this is going to achieve nothing and she should not have been paid. The people she ripped off should have.

Crass, arrogant, deceitful and dangerous.

So everyone else is lying and Belle Gibson is the only one that is truthful. just admit it YOU LIED! Disgusting pig.

Cancer took out my father, and it's shadow has crossed another family member just this week. I am LIVID.

Lying manipulative bitch.

To lie about a disease so gut wrenching and serious as cancer is an absolute outrage and travesty.

Belle Gibson should hang out with Lance Armstrong, oh the sympathy they could offer one another.

Australian Rules footballer Luke Delaney posted that his 'blood's boiling after that': 'No responsibility or empathy for thousands of REAL cancer sufferers. Absolute low life.' On reports that Gibson had been paid a tidy sum for the televised appearance, Jaala Pulford, an MP in the Victorian state government, told Twitter she was 'disgusted that Belle Gibson is still profiteering at the expense of people with cancer'. Social media began circulating an online petition, signed by more than 11,200 people, calling for Gibson's appearance payment to be handed over to cancer research instead.

'Belle Gibson is playing us for fools,' the petition said. 'She fed us false claims of cancer survival, a neglected childhood and the healing powers of organic foods. Now she continues to obtain money off her fraudulent lies … Belle Gibson was a fake who took our honest money to hear her "inspiring story", promising $300,000 would be donated to cancer charities — but not one charity received a cent from her … Belle, it may be impossible for you to undo the damage your lies created, but you can certainly start at charity donations.'

In the 2015 bestseller *So You've Been Publicly Shamed*, Welsh writer Jon Ronson explored how the ultra-modern phenomenon of social media has, in fact, spurred a resurgence of the distinctly old-world ritual of public shamings. The book tracked the harrowing tales of people whose lives had been upended by the hellfire of Twitter and Facebook damnation: Justine Sacco, a PR executive who tweeted a bad joke about AIDS in Africa; Jonah Lehrer, a pop-science author who was caught out fabricating Bob Dylan quotes; a woman named Lindsey Stone, who posted a photo of herself flipping the bird in front of a 'Silence and Respect' sign at a national cemetery. It was Ronson's contention that the punishments — huge public shamings that crushed people's careers and tarnished their names forever — often far outweighed their so-called crimes. Certainly, Belle Gibson's transgression was truly more unthinkable. It was far less forgivable than plagiarism or offensive tweets. But had the ritualistic shaming of Belle Gibson now gone too far?

When you type her name into Twitter, the torrent of abuse directed at Gibson is overwhelming. People tweeted about Gibson in English, Arabic, Italian, Spanish, French, Turkish, Japanese, Filipino. Her name is sometimes used as a synonym for fraud, with one tweet criticising Donald Trump as the Belle Gibson of politics. She was called garbage, disgusting, a 'vile human', 'charlatan', 'liar', 'con artist', and, literally, 'the worst person in the world'.

People like Belle Gibson make me sick.

What a disgusting human being.

I hope she catches something that they can't cure.

Just throw Belle Gibson in jail FFS.

Belle Gibson, you are lower than a sewer rat.

Some posts went even further. They were more vicious, more violent. Some went as far as wishing she would die:

Baseball bat to the skull is the only cure.

People like Belle Gibson should be shot. I wish her a slow death.

I don't think I've ever said this about anyone in my life, but Belle Gibson should kill herself.

Social media, it seemed, was united in its hatred of her. The venom in the attacks on Gibson was of the type usually reserved for paedophiles and war criminals. Her scam, regardless of whether she was mad or bad, was collectively deemed to be so offensive. Not just because of the lie itself, but because Gibson had played off society's better nature: she took advantage of people's trust, their sympathy. The public reaction to this deception, a deception that gave false hope to cancer sufferers, was absolutely gut-twisting. In 2015, the *Washington Post* even ranked Gibson in the top-10 *Internet Villains of the Year.*

The participatory internet was Gibson's world. It was where she had once flourished, gathered sympathy and attention, and amassed her 'community'. She was undeniably, as her publisher described her, a social-media sensation. Now the very world in which she thrived had completely turned on her. One Twitter user posted: 'I've only skimmed the surface about Belle Gibson … but it seems like she WILL be the victim if anyone on social media gets their hands on her.' Gibson was trapped, utterly drenched in shame.

If the Twitterverse was a courtroom, Gibson's attempt to mount a defence that she was a victim had failed resoundingly.

'Truth, Belle,' Tara kept imploring, 'the truth.'

'Tara, I'm trying to draw on information —'

'No, no. Don't *draw* on information,' she said. 'Just be honest.'

For many, the voiceover said, Belle Gibson was the wellness warrior: 'Her good health was the great hope for her followers, especially those battling cancer themselves. What is really worrying is how many of them may have given up conventional treatment to follow Belle's alternative path. Again, Belle, tries to dodge her responsibility.'

'But I was not an expert in anyone else's health,' Gibson said.

'Excuse me, excuse me,' Tara interjected. 'But don't be naive now. I mean, you are appealing to an incredibly vulnerable audience, incredibly vulnerable people.'

'Mm-hm.'

'You have a responsibility to make sure your story is right.'

'I'm not trying to get away with anything.' The camera cuts to Tara. She looks down, smiles, and exhales loudly. Gibson continues. 'I'm not trying to smooth over anything. It's not easy for me to be here, it's not easy for me to relive and relive and relive detail.'

'How do you think it is for the people who followed, whose heart went out to you when you wrote about how unwell you were, how well you were, your progress, your decline. These [are] people who cried for you. Have you thought about them? I know you sit here and tell me how you feel. Have you thought about how they're feeling at the moment?'

'I put them in my shoes, and I know that they're feeling the same way I feel.'

'Some of them want you to go to jail. That's how they feel.'

'I know that they feel that way — I've seen the emails, I've seen some of the comments. I'm on the receiving end of all of that, Tara. And I take responsibility for how this has unfolded.'

'Do you take responsibility for driving any people away from conventional medicine in seeking treatment for their cancer?'

'That would be really heartbreaking to me, because I never intended on doing that.'

'Do you accept that that's what you might have done.'

'I accept that might have happened.'

Towards the end of the interview, Tara appears to throw Gibson a lifeline.

'I just wonder, Belle, if — and I don't know if you're at a stage where you'll ever admit it, but — whether you just didn't know what you were getting yourself into? That you probably thought you weren't doing any harm, but that you thought you could get away with it?'

'There was nothing to get away with, Tara.'

'Oh, of course there was. There was adulation, there's sympathy, there's a community who loves you, there's huge amounts to get away with —'

'There's a community that I love.'

'You kind of were playing in a grown-up's world without realising it,' Tara continues, shaking her head. 'But it was all going to end badly.'

'It didn't need to,' Gibson said. 'Once I started to figure out where I stood and what reality actually was, and I had received the definitive "No, you do not have cancer", then that was something that I had to come to terms with. That takes a lot. And it was really traumatising, I was feeling a huge amount of grief, and —'

'Grief for not having cancer?'

'No. That I had been lied to and, um, that I felt like I had been taken for a ride. It took me a lot to unpack that. And once I was strong enough, I was ready to come out and speak with my community about it. And I had a definitive date, and that date was only ten days before the media broke it.'

No one believed her, yet the *60 Minutes* grilling was so brutal to watch — 'shooting fish in the barrel,' as one called it — that, in amongst the furore, some called for mercy:

Am I the only person who feels for Belle Gibson? It's time to leave her alone.

I have left the Belle Gibson interview feeling very, very sad. Belle Gibson is clearly not well.

When the one-year anniversary of the scandal approached, each news article, feature, or comment piece on developments big and small were still pulling big numbers, averaging between 50,000 and

100,000 readers for each story. The scandal was still being widely reported in Australia and around the world. On 5 May 2016, Gibson put up a rare post on her personal Facebook page. It was a link to a Monica Lewinsky video titled, 'The Price of Shame', a TED talk by the one-time White House intern with whom former president Bill Clinton admitted having a sexual relationship. It was about the impact of cyberbullying and online harassment.

'Leaving this here,' Gibson wrote, 'Have watched this a few times, and still just so resounding. Tread kindly. People can and do hurt deeply and that hurt can live within for a long, long time. Brave, Monica.'

20

KATE THOMAS — PART I

The scars from the surgeon's incisions on the front of Kate Thomas' body are threaded together like a patchwork quilt. Her left breast was cut off, and the muscle, fat, and blood vessels under her belly-button sucked out and sculpted to create a new one. Fourteen of the 18 lymph nodes under her left arm were cancerous, so they were cut out, too. For almost half a year, she had chemotherapy at The Alfred hospital in Melbourne. It was administered through a port in her chest the size of a 20-cent coin that was attached to a vein in her neck. The treatment made Kate vomit, faint, tire, run fevers, lose her appetite, and get ulcers in her mouth and her throat. It made water taste like salt, and food taste like nothing. Her bones throbbed. Her hair, eyebrows, and eyelashes fell out. Her skin turned dry and scaly, her eyes watered constantly, and her face puffed up. The nails on her toes rotted and fell off.

The medication Kate was prescribed forced her body into early menopause, at 35. If she's lucky enough to sleep at night, she'll wake on a mattress soaked through with sweat. She aches all over and always. Her bones are brittle: osteoporosis has stricken her spine, knees, and hips. She is at high risk of a spine fracture. In August 2016, Kate cracked a rib lifting a table. In September, she had keyhole heart surgery at the Royal Melbourne Hospital to repair a pathway damaged by the radiation. She takes hormone blockers, calcium, and Vitamin D supplements, probiotics, enzymes, painkillers, high-dose antidepressants to manage the menopause symptoms, Gabapentin for the hot flushes, and Melatonin to sleep. Every month, a nurse uses a huge needle to shoot a pellet into her stomach to decrease her oestrogen levels. All the medication has made her fingers swell. Her wedding band and the diamond engagement ring she inherited from her grandmother sit in a box at home.

This is what cancer looks like. It is devastating and debilitating and deadly. When Kate first got sick, she didn't know what the disease and its treatments could do to the human body. But she did know about Belle Gibson: the young working mother and cancer survivor who was jet-setting around the world, staying in hotels in New York and in Bali. Gibson had moved house, started a global business from the ground up, and written a cookbook — all in a year, all while she was supposedly sick.

Kate is the kind of person you can't help but like instantly. She is sweet, honest, and funny. Her blue-green eyes are big and bright, and they seem larger still behind her tortoise-shell glasses. She is a vegan, and she has several tattoos, all covered by clothes except for one, on her left elbow, of a butterfly and the circle of life. Kate first met Gibson at a party in St Kilda in 2013, where Gibson made a speech about her cancer and the lifestyle changes she'd made. Kate was inspired by her — as so many were — and when she went home that night she downloaded The Whole Pantry app. She later bought a copy of Gibson's spinoff cookbook by the same name, and started following the social-media starlet online, watching on from afar as her star continued to rise. On 29 July 2014, Kate logged onto Instagram and saw a long post in her feed; it was from Gibson, announcing to her 200,000-plus followers that her cancer had spread. It was the one in which she announced her cancer had metastasised from her brain, infiltrating her liver, her spleen, her cervix, her uterus:

> With frustration and ache in my heart // my beautiful, gamechanging community, it hurts me to find space tonight to let you all know with love and strength that I've been diagnosed with a third and forth [sic] cancer. One is secondary and the other is primary. I have cancer in my blood, spleen, brain, uterus, and liver. I am hurting …

This can't be happening, Kate said to herself. Tears welled in her eyes and ran down her cheeks. She typed Gibson a message of heartfelt support. Then she started thinking about herself, and that made her cry some more.

Kate had been diagnosed with breast cancer in February 2014. She was 34 years old and had been married to her husband, Nik, for just a year. She had been managing a nice little café not far from her apartment, and was about to open her own dog daycare business. Then one day, at the end of summer, just as she was undressing to take a shower, she felt it: a small, egg-shaped swelling, a lump, on the upper outer part of her breast. Kate went to her GP, who told her she needed to see a specialist right away. Kate had tickets to see Dolly Parton play at Rod Laver Arena that night. She'd been looking forward to it for months. She didn't get to go.

Three days later, the specialist examined her. Then she performed a needle biopsy. It hurt like hell. The specialist was frank; she told Kate it was serious, and that there was a reason for her to be concerned. Kate felt as though all the oxygen had been sucked out of the room. She wasn't prepared to hear that. She was young, and had always taken care of herself. She had a clean diet, didn't smoke, barely ever drank. But her worst fears were soon her reality.

Her voice quivered as she told Nik over the phone. 'Um,' she said. 'I think I've got cancer.'

The clinic was in East Melbourne, not far from Nik's office on Victoria Street, where he worked for an insurance company, so he was there quickly. Nik took Kate out for dinner before they went home. That was Friday, Valentine's Day. On Monday, the results were back. They were conclusive: breast cancer, stage three.

In Australia, the US, and the UK, about one in eight women will be diagnosed with breast cancer in her lifetime. The type of cancer Kate has strikes almost 800 women under the age of 40 every year in Australia. Like Kate, these women, often in their 20s and 30s, are planning to start a family or are forging their career paths. The National Breast Cancer Foundation says younger women are typically diagnosed with more aggressive breast cancers than older women. These cancers are the type that are more likely to spread, to return, and to kill.

Kate stopped sleeping properly. She lay in bed awake. Her world felt upended. Her fear of dying was overwhelming and often unstoppable. When sleep didn't come, and the worries filled her head, Kate would scroll through her iPhone, breezing, aimlessly and with barely a pause, through streams of crafted Instagram photos. She liked the beautiful photos; the flattering filters; the shots of interesting clothes. But Nik soon noticed something change. There had been a shift. She wasn't doing that anymore; now she was reading things more intently. She was engrossed, captivated by someone, or by something. Kate started to talk about the amazing Belle Gibson.

'To see that she had gone through this, but had done it the

natural way, was inspiring,' Kate recalls. 'She gave hope to people like me that maybe we didn't have to put ourselves through such intense treatment. Maybe we could survive.'

Kate Thomas met Nik Donaldson late one night in 2006, at a live-music club called Ding Dong Lounge, which is upstairs in a lane in Melbourne's Chinatown. Nik was a drummer in an indie-rock band. He was handsome, with swept hair, and conspicuously cool. Kate sidled up to him and plucked the beer from his hand. She took a sip, and told him she was keeping it.

'I used to be quite forward,' Kate grins, and glances over at Nik. 'He had no choice in it.'

Their wedding was stylish and small. Kate wore a white 1950s day dress that she designed herself; it was full at the bottom and buttoned up with a Peter Pan collar. She had crimson high-heels and a bright-red rose in her hair, tightly woven. Nik was dressed in the Teddy Boy style — rubber-sole rockabilly creepers, a white shirt, drape jacket, and Western bow tie. His three groomsmen — his two younger brothers and his best mate — wore the same. They called it their 'Vintage Rockabilly Vegan Wedding'. It had a mid-century high-tea theme; Kate baked all the cupcakes and scones and lamingtons herself. The food was served on vintage crockery, and laid out on lace tablecloths. Kate arrived in a light-pink classic EK Holden. She had one bridesmaid, her friend, Sarah, and walked down the aisle to Amy Winehouse's *Between the Cheats*. The 40 guests at the ceremony were mostly Nik's family, who had flown over from New Zealand. Nik's parents, both celebrants, married the couple. Their first dance was around the corner, at the Napier Hotel, just the two of them.

Nik is a slick rocker who tours with two bands — 'he's good,' says

Kate, '*real good*' — but there's nothing brash about him. He is soft-spoken and thoughtful, gentle and warm-hearted. He is extremely well-read and considered in his views, and he always listens with undivided attention.

He sits beside Kate at an outdoor table, at their local café, overlooking a public reserve, and orders two espressos. Their French bulldog, Brando, is perched on his lap. Nik internalises his fears and his sadness. Sometimes, it feels like he has been slugged in the stomach, or that they are floating about like it is all a bad dream. But he tries to be a calming presence for Kate; he tries to be her rock. He tries to stay focused on what the next battle is, and the next appointment, and, during Kate's chemotherapy, his life's mission became helping her through it. He bought books about it, and held her hair back when was sick from the side effects. But then the second round of chemo began, and things became harder than either of them could imagine.

'I can't do this,' Kate wept one night, utterly drained and hurting everywhere. 'I can't.'

Kate quickly made up her mind. It wasn't a discussion. The thought of vomiting for months on end terrified her. She wanted to go down a path that mimicked Gibson's, and fight the cancer with nutrition, healthy living, organic juices, and Gerson Therapy. She was now spending hours on the internet, reading and researching recipes and regimens, the clinics in Germany, the coffee enemas. Then she bought herself a cold-pressed juicer. Nik was almost certain that his wife was going to stray from conventional medicine entirely. One night, his gentle tone changed. His face flushed, and his expression became stony. He looked straight into Kate's eyes and said forcefully: '*You're not doing it.*'

He wasn't going to let a 'hippie with a juicing machine and an Instagram page' undercut years of medical progress that could give his wife the best chance of staying alive. He just wasn't.

'If you want to eat certain foods or want to go organic, no problem,' he told her, 'but there is no way you are not going to do conventional medicine. You are going to do your chemo, and you're going to do your radiation program like they said, because these are doctors, and these are the people who know as much about cancer as we can.'

Kate was taken aback. She really didn't know what to say.

'He just said, "No" … you're sticking with it,' Kate recalls. 'I was a bit shocked that he was so firm. He is usually so supportive of anything I do. But I think that this came out of fear.'

In the days that followed, Nik was scared. He wasn't convinced the woman he loved was hearing him. He called on his mother, Janine Donaldson, a nurse, to speak with Kate on Skype from her home in New Zealand. Nik was born on the South Island city of Dunedin, but he has lost his Kiwi accent. Both his parents were missionaries with the Salvation Army, and, when he was a boy, they took him to live in Zambia, where he went to primary school and spent much of his childhood, before returning to New Zealand and attending high school in Auckland. Janine spent 10 years all up working in Africa, so she was familiar with many natural remedies and their varied benefits. She has seen healing from the use of natural resources at first hand. But she has also seen it fail, and has watched on helplessly as people remained stubbornly resistant to conventional medical intervention that could have made a difference. On the Skype call, Janine was alarmed at Kate's constant references to Gibson — some girl she had never heard of.

'You've got to do what your doctors say, Kate,' she urged. 'You are going to get through this.' She promised her they would do it together.

'Kate is my daughter-in-law after three sons,' Janine says in an email from her apartment in Beckenham, in London's south-east, where she and her husband now live. 'She is precious to me. I simply did not want to risk her life, I did not want her to lose her. I relayed this to her in no uncertain terms. I paused sometimes to think how pushy I was, yet I couldn't help myself.'

Janine bought a plane ticket and flew to Melbourne, to stay with Nik and Kate, and to help Kate through the chemo. She went to almost every session with her daughter-in-law. And back at home, she sat with Kate on the cold tiles on the bathroom floor. Kate vomited and groaned in pain as the chemicals coursed through her body. Her face was chalky and sweat-soaked. She thought she was dying, and begged Janine to take her to the emergency room. Janine gently rubbed her back, and said some prayers.

'I hated the way through the treatment her lovely hair fell out,' Janine recalls. 'I grieved about the lousy way she continually felt, and I continue to grieve over the nasty scars on her body. The big question is, did I do the right thing by her? Did I push too hard? Would an alternative have been better? Was my advice worthy to be taken? I can't honestly answer that and I have never asked Kate. I feel enormous guilt over not helping her enough.'

Nik and Janine urged Kate to listen to her oncologist, a man who bluntly described the proposed treatment regime as the 'hamburger with the lot'. What this metaphor meant was that Kate's body would become unrecognisable. But they convinced her it was the right thing to do. Kate has had 38 rounds of radiation, five months of chemotherapy, and a mastectomy — and even still, she will have to take a cocktail of medication every day for the next 10 years. Her chances of being alive in a decade are fifty-fifty.

–21–

HOPING FOR A MIRACLE CURE

At the little cemetery on Rarotonga, the largest of the Cook Islands north of New Zealand, the graves of the dead slipped off the coast and were swallowed by the sea. Sixty or so headstones remain, marking the final resting place for the cancer patients — Australians, most of them; desperate, all of them — who travelled here in the late 1970s hoping for a cure. The rows of graves on this eroding parcel of land are wedged between the break and the one runway servicing the small island's airport. Officially, this place is called Nikao Cemetery. But to locals, it's Brych Yard, named after Milan Brych, a self-styled cancer therapist who gave false hope to the terminally ill and left a trail of bodies across the Pacific.

Brych (pronounced Brick) came to New Zealand in 1968 as a refugee from communist Czechoslovakia. He claimed to be a doctor, and soon got a job as a cancer therapist in the oncology unit at Auckland Hospital. In the early 1970s, he treated terminal cancer patients with what he said was immunotherapy. His treatments were said to consist of multiple injections of a serum taken from the patient's blood, although critics believed he used nothing more than standard chemotherapy and high doses of steroids, which can lead to short-term improvements and mask the severity of some conditions. Nevertheless, Brych's patients, all whom faced imminent death, were staying alive longer. Before long, stories were spreading about the exotic young doctor in Ward Eleven who was working miracles. Brych courted the spotlight. He invited the media to meet with his dewy-eyed patients. 'The Doctor They Call God,' one newspaper called him in a headline.

Brych was a short man with a wide forehead and dark, receding hair. He had a stiff, measured walk, and was supremely confident and flamboyant: he liked bold shirts and white suits, and wore big, square glasses. He was flashy, and earned a reputation as a playboy. Brych revelled in being *the* in-demand cancer specialist of the day. But as his profile grew, so too did questions about his methods. When challenged to produce evidence that his treatment worked, Brych always baulked. He refused to run a double-blind trial, and never published any findings to support his work. If his treatment was so successful, *why wouldn't he share it?* Opponents labelled him a quack and a charlatan, and, eventually, medical authorities discovered he was a fraud; it turned out he'd never studied medicine and was, in fact, in a Czech prison for robbery at the time he claimed to have earned his qualification as a doctor. An inquiry later found there was no evidence he had ever treated any of his patients with immunotherapy.

Brych had been outed as an imposter, but this didn't seem to make a difference. He had a devoted following: patients who had outlived the terminal prognosis they were given by other doctors. Brych was celebrated and fiercely defended by these patients and their families. Like advocates for most questionable cancer treatments, Brych's apologists argued he was doing something that nobody else would do. They clung to the idea that there was some kind of conspiracy at work — a cure that the government kept secret, or which threatened pharmaceutical companies' profits. It didn't matter that he wasn't a doctor; he had the answer, and he should not be stopped from administering his life-saving treatment. Brych's chief supporter was the late Queensland premier Joh Bjelke-Petersen, who wanted him to set up a cancer clinic in the city of Brisbane. Doctors railed against the government's plan to make sure it never happened.

Brych left New Zealand, and moved to the nearby Cook Islands, and it was on the rugged island of Rarotonga that he headed up the local cancer unit. Hundreds of patients were lured from Australia. They called him Doctor, paying roughly $10,000 each for his treatment, which they described as a six-month regimen of drips and injections. Many of them died. There were no autopsies on Rarotonga, and, as was the custom, the dead were buried within 24 hours in the little cemetery overlooking the ocean. Over the years, about a dozen graves have slipped off the remote island and have been washed away, their crumbling headstones left stranded on the shore. The remaining ones are relics to the infinite desperation felt by the people who once came here asking for help.

The Milan Brych case is one of the most high-profile cancer scams in recent history, but it is by no means unique. Self-proclaimed healers and so-called alternative practitioners have always deceived the sick and the vulnerable, selling a swathe of potions and promises. Cancer patients top the list of desperate people ripe to be lured into this flourishing cottage industry. These shysters who prey on them have touted the curative powers of everything from supplements to spirituality. They've sold salt water and herbal tea and juice, and high-dose intravenous vitamins, hash oil, flax seeds, and mistletoe. They have pedalled their cure du jour in varying forms of special alkalising diets and detoxes. And prescribed black salve, and laetrile, which is found in the seeds of some fruit, such as apricot pits. They have pushed homeopathic remedies and extreme hyperthermia treatment, and magnet, ozone, and electrical therapies, and crystals and colonics and hypnosis.

In one particularly disturbing case, two dozen terminal cancer patients died after rejecting conventional medicine and paying tens of thousands of dollars for a so-called miracle cure. In 2005, in Perth, Australia, four patients were dead within two weeks of beginning the treatment, which included intravenous infusions containing laetrile, caesium chloride, and an industrial solvent called DSMO. The cocktail of drugs was administered in a suburban home at the direction of disgraced Austrian doctor Hellfried Sartori, who had previously been jailed in the US for practising medicine without a licence. It was promoted as having a 95 to 98 per cent cure rate if the patient truly believed in the treatment, and was sold as 'natural' and 'safe'. West Australian deputy state coroner Evelyn Vicker ruled it was neither. 'It requires high doses of industrially manufactured substances and is manifestly unsafe,' she wrote in 2012. 'There is no doubt [Sartori] now perceives families desperate enough to turn to him, as experimental subjects who will pay for a chance, any chance, to survive.'

Many, many thousands of patients have trawled the globe in search of a magic bullet, travelling to clinics in Europe, to markets in Asia, and to the neon-lit streets of Tijuana. What Brych shares with his nefarious alumni of snake-oil salesmen is a trail of exploits targeting the desperate and the dying with the expensive lure of false hope.

Andrew Kaye walks briskly down a narrow corridor to his sixth-floor office in his wing of the hospital, and closes the door behind him. Andrew is busy. He gestures towards the couch opposite a wall of shelves stocked with encyclopedias and medical books, models of skulls, framed photos, plaques, and awards. He sits, cross-legged, in front of the shelves, and starts talking about cancer scams even before we get to the couch.

'The big problem with all this,' Andrew begins, 'and why I'm talking to you — because otherwise I wouldn't be — is that people are in the most vulnerable situation when they're told they have got an incurable cancer.'

Andrew doesn't hold back what he thinks. He is the first to admit that he can be a bit tactless. But he has a warm manner. He seems discerning and caring; the type of person you would want to tell you if you had a tumour growing in your brain.

'If you come to me with a malignant brain cancer that has recurred, I would have to say there is no way we are going to cure you,' he says. Then he says it again: 'There is no way. We may be able to help your life a bit, we *may* be able to. But we cannot cure you.

'But if you go to someone who says there is a very small chance you can be cured, well, people will grasp at that, and they'll sell their homes. And this happens over and over and over and over again through the whole range of cancers.

'It's an enormous issue.'

Andrew is one of Australia's leading neurosurgeons. He is based at the Royal Melbourne Hospital in Parkville, Melbourne. Over his long career, Andrew has come across many different types of cancer scams. Everyone who works in oncology has. It's an unfortunate part of the landscape. The oncologists we spoke to said much the same thing: patients generally don't turn down life-saving or curative treatment. But, if the cancer comes back, if it spreads, if it is terminal, patients and their families will search for alternatives. Studies show that the use of complementary or alternative treatment is widespread among cancer patients (alternative therapies are used instead of conventional treatment, while complementary therapies are used in conjunction with conventional treatment). Tertiary-educated young women are the most likely to seek them out.

'The biggest problem we've had is people going onto these "special treatments" instead of what is conventional, best treatment,' Andrew says. 'Sometimes people are lured into cancer scams because they have a distrust of the medical profession, and sometimes that distrust is justified. But, mainly, it's the futility of the diagnosis, and the hope for something better. Commonly, they have had a [conventional] treatment, and then the cancer comes back, and then they go off and search for something else.

'But it's not going to help, and it could make it worse, and they're going to spend a lot of money.'

The scams, Andrew says, run the full gamut. Often, they will have a very thin basis in science but, when scrutinised, the treatment simply doesn't hold up. The person selling the therapy is usually a real salesperson, too; they'll always over-promise, something that doctors are cautious to do. But the real test of it, says Andrew and his colleagues, is the cost of the so-called miracle treatment. *Who is going to make a buck out of this?*

In Belle Gibson's case, where she herself claimed to be suffering from cancer, something more complicated was at play. She chose the scariest disease in one of its most aggressive forms. In doing so, she played off the public's better nature. Australian ethicist Julie Crews explains that Gibson's story was taken at face value because people reason — consciously or unconsciously — that a sick person is also a truthful person. 'Belle Gibson took it to a whole other level,' Julie says. 'What's really interesting is that a lot of the people who were taken in were young women. I'm interested in the principal question: why are young women willing to listen to someone like Belle Gibson or Jess Ainscough instead of the scientists who know what they are talking about?'

Before becoming an academic, Julie worked in the Australian Competition and Consumer Commission's small-business division. She has been exposed to a lot of different types of scams. 'Belle is no different from the countless potential fraudsters out there willing to deceive people to make money,' Julie says. 'Unlike being "done over" by someone selling, say, a dodgy car where you lose money, "cancer gurus" play to a vulnerable group who may abandon evidence-based medicine for the hope being peddled [by] unproven alternative therapies.'

Julie lists example after example of health scammers. Some have written books, or work as health coaches, or have 'cured their cancer'. They are similar in a couple of distinct ways. 'They all just cherry-pick the truth,' Julie says, 'and there's always these tenuous links, like, *I was given six months to live and now look at me, I'm cured.*'

Julie has used Belle Gibson as a case study in her classes. She explains that snake-oil merchants have always existed, but the way in which they operate has become much more sophisticated. It's not a face-to-face transaction anymore — victims are targeted online. She asks her undergraduate students what an appropriate response is when someone like Gibson makes such extreme claims. 'Number one,' Julie says, 'is verify the facts. But you'd be very surprised by what people say. Social media is one of the main ways that young people get their information now, and even when presented with the facts, it doesn't seem to matter. Opinion has morphed into fact.'

Another respected oncologist in Melbourne is Mark Rosenthal. He explains how patient-blaming is at the heart of many alternative treatments on the market. 'Patients are told: "You lived a dirty life to get cancer, or you've done something wrong, or your psychology was wrong so you deserved to get it."' This is what Mark says underpins the sales pitch. He isn't talking about diseases with known causative links to lifestyle habits, such as smoking and lung cancer. He's talking about the concept that a person who has cancer is somehow responsible for getting the disease. From there, he explains, it's not a far leap to another facile concept: that conquering cancer is dependent on the patient's willingness, or desire, or positive attitude. 'Take, for example, an aggressive brain cancer, and someone says to you that it can be conquered. Well, no, you can't conquer it. So somehow you've failed because your cancer grew and you're dying,' Mark says. 'Once you've got an incurable cancer, it's incurable. This notion of war, battle … I have to dissuade people that it's a "fight", because if it's a terminal cancer, that is a "fight" they are going to lose. We have to try to counterbalance that idea that the patient is to blame.'

Mark is the director of a clinical trials unit, and a senior oncologist who has worked across neuro-oncology, prostate, and kidney cancer. He has seen first-hand how cancer treatments have improved and become more targeted over the years. More is known about the disease now than ever before. But as the medical understanding of cancer improves, he says, the community's thinking about the disease has become more irrational. We are becoming less trusting of the science. Simple remedies are far more appealing than complex discussions about a terminal diagnosis. Or mortality. Mark now pre-empts conversations with patients before they ask him. Because they will ask him. And he's about as blunt as he can be.

'I say: there will be lots of people with well-meaning advice, telling you to eat this, drink that, do this, don't do that. It's all bullshit. I wish there was magic, but there is no magic. I have this conversation every day of the week, I've done it for 15 years. If there was magic, and I didn't have to have this terrible conversation, I'd be using magic. If standing in a bucket of manure was going to make a difference, you'd be standing in a bucket of manure, and there would be a long line of people out the door behind you. It doesn't work. If drinking a glass of orange juice makes you feel better, or coffee enemas or shark cartilage make you feel better, then fine, but if it was going to help treat your cancer, then we would be doing it. Meditating, great. Yoga, great. Healthy diet, great. But if it sounds too good to be true, it's too good to be true. And if it sounds crazy, it's crazy.'

One of Mark's patients died on an aeroplane en route home from Germany after undergoing experimental cancer therapy. That's the worst outcome he's come across involving an alternative medicine. But he points out that the people who prey on the sick are not confined to the shadows. He says some conventional doctors also sell false hope and have pushed questionable treatments. One of Brych's biggest supporters was a Melbourne GP who referred his cancer patients to Rarotonga. Mark says there are surgeons in Australia (he won't name them) who charge small fortunes to perform operations that may not be worthwhile. But that begs the question, *What is worthwhile?* Is it an extra two or three weeks of life? Or six or 12 months? Another of Mark's patients died in intensive care after having an operation that he recommended against. That's the worst outcome he's come across involving conventional cancer medicine.

Mark holds up his hands as though they're a set of scales, raising one as he lowers the other. 'I do this all the time,' he says. 'The question is always: how much good can we do, versus how much harm can we do? It's about balance. The balance of why we choose treatments, and why we don't use treatments.' Mark knows to the percentage point the chances of his patients surviving their incurable cancer for six months, 12 months, five years, and even 10 years. But he tries not to put circles on calendars. Rather, he tells his patients that every person with incurable cancer is different, that their illness is unique, and that time will tell.

Mark also knows the chances that his patients have of benefiting from a certain type of medicine, compared to how likely they are to be harmed by it. That is the fundamental difference between conventional and alternative medicine. Doctors have to rely on the best available research and scientific evidence to assess, diagnose, and treat their patients. Alternative medicine, on the other hand, is often based on anecdotal evidence: wisdom passed down from generations, expertise garnered from case studies, word-of-mouth endorsements, and, increasingly, endorsements on Google, Wikipedia, and Instagram. This does not mean that all alternative medicines are useless. But most haven't been assessed for their efficacy and safety in double-blind, randomised, controlled trials. That means their scientific basis has not been established. There has been no rigorous evaluation by ethics committees, no oversight from regulatory bodies, and, therefore, no clarity over what the patient is actually getting. The point of relying on scientific evidence is to mitigate and clearly communicate the risk of harm. If we don't, how can we know what risk was considered before one course of medical treatment was recommended over another? *What risk of harm did Gibson consider when she gave health advice? What risk of harm did Apple and Penguin consider when they promoted her miraculous cancer-survival story?*

Cancer is complicated. It is not a single disease. And it has been around for thousands of years. The path to getting a drug funded, trialled, approved, and peer reviewed is tortuous for a reason. The alternative is the equivalent to an online classified. *Complementary* therapies, on the other hand, can be beneficial for cancer patients. But scams such as Gibson's give all forms of unconventional treatment a bad name; they widen the yawning divide between conventional medicine and complementary therapies that are proven to actually help patients.

Mark doesn't criticise the terminal patients who don't heed

his advice and go searching for something else. There's a cultural expectation, he says, to try everything possible, as futile as that might be. Sometimes it's not even being driven by the patient themselves; it's pushed for by their families. Of course, the alternatives are always sold as something that puts the power back into the hands of the patient, giving them autonomy and just a glimmer of hope. When he describes these patients, he uses words like brave, courageous, grateful, and gracious. He says they deserve a quiet, peaceful death. Often, though, in these cases, that doesn't happen.

'The conversation about "no more treatment" is a really tough conversation,' Mark says. 'There should be an acceptance and a recognition that someone is dying. It's a special time, not an easy time, but a special time. It can be a profound time: things are said that need to be said, things are done, patients resolve matters, plan for their family, and settle their affairs. And I think with a lot of these treatments — you might go overseas, you might try certain things, spend a lot of money, put in a lot of effort — you lose that time. The time that should be spent holding hands, talking, comforting each other. That's lost.'

There is just one headstone in Brych Yard that bears the Star of David. It belongs to Nathan Steinkoler. He died on Rarotonga on 12 September 1977. 'I still don't feel like I'm over it, to be honest with you,' his son, Leon, says through tears, the first time he speaks to us about Milan Brych. 'When I think about what Milan Brych did to me and my family … I think that he robbed us.' Leon Steinkoler was 19 years old when his father died at Brych's island clinic. He's now about to turn 60.

Nathan, a Polish Jew, was a Holocaust survivor. His father and two brothers were murdered in Auschwitz; his mother died in the

Lodz ghetto; his sister was tortured, and worse. Nathan came to Melbourne in 1950, and started a delicatessen on Nicholson Street in Footscray. He worked hard, and valued an education for his children, Leon and his older sister, Adele. But he was a damaged person and a very private man; he didn't talk about the war or the camps. In the late 1970s, when he was diagnosed with mesothelioma, a cancer of the lung caused by asbestos exposure, a Melbourne doctor referred him to Brych. Leon was about to sit his second-year exams to become a pharmacist, and his dad wanted him to stay at home and study. Leon remembers the last words his father spoke to him at the airport. 'He said, "Don't worry, I'll be back soon,"' Leon recalls. Within a month, Nathan was dead. There were no embalming facilities on the island, and so his body was buried the next day.

Leon has many unanswered questions about his father's treatment, about why he deteriorated so quickly when he seemed well just weeks earlier, but he understands that the disease was terminal. It's *how* his father died that haunts him still; how the final moments of his life were stolen from the family — precious moments when, sometimes, the dying say things that have gone unsaid for so long, moments that could have been life-changing for the next generation that inherited the trauma of war. Leon has seen it before. Australia has one of the largest Holocaust survivor populations per capita outside Israel. He was raised in Melbourne, home to more survivors than anywhere else in the country. He's watched as a generation of Jews tattooed with Nazi ink has passed away.

'It's that critical time that was taken from us, that time when maybe he would have opened up, maybe he would have told me his story, like other survivors did as they neared closer to death,' Leon says. 'Dad was going to die, I know that, but he didn't die with us. I've spent years trying to piece together bits and pieces, and it's very hard because my father never told me anything, and then in the end he was taken, and I'm left feeling empty.'

Among the death records on Rarotonga is that of a young dancer from Melbourne, a farmer, and a lecturer. Christal Barker, 36, a mother of three, died on 7 June 1977. Joan Cossar, who had eight children, died four days later, and 21-year-old Christopher Homan passed away that same week. Thomas Fowler, 50, and Elisa Maree King, 9, both died in November. The youngest of Brych's patients, five-year-old Jarred Nutt, who had a tumour in his head, died in the arms of his parents, Sonja and John, two days before Christmas.

Gloria Walker was a primary-school teacher in a Queensland farming region called the Darling Downs. She was diagnosed with advanced breast cancer when she was 35 years old. It was December 1976, a time when breast-cancer therapy was still in its infancy and when Brych was being hailed as a miracle worker. Gloria and her husband, Bob, flew to Rarotonga from Brisbane, and Gloria was treated at Brych's clinic. At first, she responded well. Gloria sent her daughters a letter. She told her three girls she was looking forward to coming home; she'd bought them some little souvenirs on the island. In another letter, to her sister, Gloria wrote that she was 'on the mend'. But after her fifth round of therapy, her condition suddenly deteriorated. Gloria died on Easter Sunday in March 1978. A week later, Bob returned to Australia without his wife, and collected his three girls from boarding school. 'Brych was huge news at the time,' says Cate, the middle daughter, now in her 50s. 'But it was just a scam, a scam to make money out of terminally ill cancer patients. These were desperate people who were taken advantage of in the most cruel way.' Cate's father told her that Brych had cried with him after Gloria died; he was apparently upset because the cancer had been 'cured' — he claimed Gloria had succumbed to a blood clot caused by a drip administered before she got to the island. Her father believed him.

Like many other Australians who flew to Rarotonga in search of a cure, Gloria died in pain, in a foreign place, far away from her children. There was no chance for goodbyes, and there was no funeral service. For decades, all that was left was a deteriorating grave in an overgrown, neglected cemetery. That upset Cate so much that she spent many years leading the effort to preserve and restore the island graveyard where her mother is buried. Such is the importance of death and a final resting place that she's come to know many of the families who lost loved ones at the hands of Milan Brych.

Not long after Nathan and Gloria were buried, Brych moved to the US, to California, where he started plying his trade again. This time, he added even more to his list of fake credentials: an honorary degree from Cambridge University, and claims to have treated Betty Ford and Happy Rockefeller. Business was as lucrative as ever: he drove a Rolls-Royce silver shadow, and lived in a Bel Air mansion.

On 15 September 1980, Brych was paid a visit. An undercover agent from the California Board of Medical Quality Assurance had been sent to meet him at a clinic in the eastern suburbs of Los Angeles. The agent was perfectly healthy, but told Brych that he had aggressive lung cancer. Brych took a blood sample from the agent, confirmed his cancer diagnosis, and promised the young man a cure. He prescribed a six-stage treatment using a special serum from Europe that would target and destroy the tumour. It would be shipped to the US, and it would cost $60,000. A week later, when the agent returned and paid the first instalment, $9,600 in cash, Brych was arrested. The 'serum', it turned out, was a common chemotherapy drug that, at the time, cost about $10 a vial.

Brych went down, convicted of numerous offences, including grand theft, practising medicine without a license, and selling a fake cancer cure. During his trial, he was described as a callous conman who preyed on terminally ill cancer patients. Superior Court judge David Aisenson said the crime targeted victims who were particularly vulnerable. Speaking after the court case, Lee Harris, the then LA district attorney, was asked if he could understand how Brych's victims could be sucked in. 'Certainly,' he replied, 'there were certainly people that testified for the defence, for Mr Brych in this proceeding, that spoke very highly of him, believing in good faith that they had been cured of cancer, when in fact, in certain instances, there was no evidence that they ever suffered from cancer, or if they had a malignancy, it was a low-grade malignancy characteristic of long-term survival.' Brych was sentenced to six years' jail, but released after three. Upon his release and deportation from the US, he was reported to be in Switzerland, and, most recently, the United Kingdom. It is unknown where he is now. If Brych is still alive, he would be in his late 70s.

On 5 May 2015, the tabloids in Britain reported that a young mother from Brighton had died after returning from a cancer clinic in Tijuana, Mexico. Samantha Beaven had been diagnosed with cervical cancer when she was pregnant with her second daughter. The primary-school teaching assistant had gone to doctors complaining of bleeding and cramps, but her symptoms were initially dismissed as part of the pregnancy.

Then, contraction-like pains started at 26 weeks. An internal exam in hospital found something on her cervix which, two days later, was confirmed as cancer. The plan was to try and make it to 30 weeks before scheduling a Caesarean and full hysterectomy, but, days later, Samantha woke up to find her waters had broken. Her second daughter, Daisy, was born the same day, in late October 2013, weighing just 1 kg.

The prognosis at that point was that the cancer could be

fought with chemotherapy and radiation, which Samantha started immediately. But then, in early 2014, Samantha developed a cough. It didn't go away after a couple of rounds of antibiotics, so an X-ray was ordered. The GP called back the same day. The cancer was now in her lungs. It was terminal.

Samantha married her husband, Alex. Their daughters Bracken, six, and baby Daisy were bridesmaids. Six months later, Samantha had a seizure. More tests revealed there were 30 to 40 tumours in her brain. She was given six months to live. Samantha was treated with cannabis oil and five sessions of palliative radiotherapy to the head. And then, she and her husband learnt about a clinic in Mexico, a city where dozens of clinics sell unconventional, unproven, and controversial cancer therapies. The family sold off their possessions, and launched a fundraiser so they could fly to Tijuana in late February 2015.

Samantha and her husband stayed there for 10 weeks, spending US$100,000 on the treatment. Then, days after returning home to the UK, Samantha died from pneumonia. She was 29 years old. The announcement on the family's Facebook page about her death said it was a lung infection, 'not the cancer', that killed her. The tabloids referred to the experimental treatment, called hypothermia treatment, as a 'pioneering' cancer therapy.

About 18 months after her death, we asked Samantha's husband, Alex, a stage builder, how he now felt about the treatment. 'The treatment, the respect, and the love from all the doctors and nurses was fantastic, they cared so much,' he told us. 'They made daily visits to people's apartments if they required it. Or even just to say hello. I strongly believe that Sam was cancer-free and feeling good after her treatment. Sadly, she caught pneumonia from the cold/air conditioning from the plane on the way home.'

He also said that two days after arriving in Tijuana, Samantha had a full body PET scan that showed her brain was cancer-free. 'The high dose of oil was working,' he said. We asked Alex for copies of the scan, so we could get them examined by an oncologist. He said he had them, but they were stored and locked away.

Hope is a difficult thing to define. Australian author Juliette O'Brien, whose cancer-specialist doctor father died of a brain tumour in 2009, wrote about it in *This is Gail*, a book about her mother's life during her husband's illness and after his death. She uses a graph showing patient survival rates for glioblastoma to capture this acute human emotion that drives us to do the extraordinary.

'Along the y-axis,' Juliette writes, 'is the number of patients still alive, and along the x-axis is time. As the curve moves from left to right, it plunges from high to low. It sweeps through milestones — three months since diagnosis, six months, one year, two years — falling towards the x-axis and illustrating fewer and fewer survivors. The curve falls to a place just above the straight black line. But it never quite reaches it. A small gap remains between the curve and the axis.

'This is where hope lives.'

22

JUDGEMENT DAY

A young government lawyer, Peter Tziotis, waited at the rectangular bench at the front of courtroom 6A in the Federal Court in Melbourne. It was just after ten o'clock on the morning of 15 March 2017. He was wearing a dark suit, a pale shirt, and a purple-and-white-striped tie. The chair at the defence table across from him was empty, just as it had been for the whole trial. Outside the building, cameras were set up on the footpath on William Street, and reporters were preparing for live crosses, hoping a judgement would land in time for the midday news.

Tziotis's exact job title was solicitor to the director of Consumer Affairs Victoria. He worked a few city blocks away, on the nineteenth floor of a large high-rise called Southern Cross Tower, on Exhibition Street. Over the past two years, staff from his office had been sending letters to Belle Gibson, and to Apple, and to Penguin. They were not so much letters as legal warrants; warrants that meant the recipients had to turn over reams of their internal documents to Consumer Affairs investigators. They demanded to see it all: emails, photographs, footage, discs, advertising material, invoices, receipts, contracts, scribbled notes, sales figures — everything that had anything to do with Gibson's charity and cancer claims.

Inside Southern Cross Tower, months were spent mining for details and meticulously building a case against the young woman. At the end of it all, Tziotis had to compile all the relevant information into two mammoth affidavits, more than 1,500 pages long, which contained every shred of evidence that was going to be used in court. Then he built the Statement of Claim, setting out, line by line, in painstaking detail, why Gibson and her business should be found guilty of multiple contraventions of consumer laws.

Since *The Age* and *The Australian* broke the earliest news stories on Gibson, in March 2015, she had been dragged through one of the biggest trials-by-media in a very long time. The first articles took investigative legwork and methodical fact-checking. But in the world of 24/7 digital news, media outlets all over the globe can pick up the story and run with it, too, sharing in the traffic, so long as there is a token degree of attribution to the original newsbreaker. Type 'reportedly' into Google News and you might think it's one of the most-used words in the news business: *Prime Minister reportedly to fast-track new laws*; *Police officer reportedly killed in shooting*. In essence, it's a convention that relieves the journalists who are told to follow up other reporters' stories from having to take the same steps of confirming information. And it means news stories like these ones can multiply far more quickly: *Belle Gibson reportedly solicited donations but failed to pass them on*; *Belle Gibson has reportedly admitted she may not have been suffering cancer at all*.

Of course, governments can never make a case as fast as the media can. The threshold for running a news article is far lower than the threshold for authorities to lay charges. Authorities need to do things more slowly and bureaucratically, regardless of the scale of the public's interest. But, just three days after *The Age*'s first story, Consumer Affairs sent a letter to Gibson to note that it had been following media coverage, and to advise her that it was an offence to solicit donations without being registered. It asked her for more details on the nature of her appeals, and gave her seven days to respond. By the next month, the long process of laying the groundwork for the *real* trial of Belle Gibson had begun.

One of Tziotis's colleagues at Consumer Affairs was a public servant named Hayden Bellis. An inspector in the department's legal services branch, Bellis was told to start making inquiries into Belle Gibson. He was handed a complaint about Gibson's fundraising activities that had been lodged by the Asylum Seeker Resource Centre, one of the charities we had alerted about Gibson's misleading use of their name in fundraising appeals.

The first thing Bellis did was buy a copy of *The Whole Pantry* cookbook from the Readings website. It cost $35. He instructed another member of his team, who had an Android phone, to download the app from Google Play. It cost $2.99. He told him to conduct a review of the app, and to take screenshots that might end up being relevant. Two days later, Bellis ran Gibson's name through the Australian Securities and Investments Commission database, and pulled the records he needed. Then, on 24 April, he wrote Gibson a letter: he wanted copies of the company's bank-account statements going back to the day she went into business. The following week, Gibson replied with the details of the company's two ANZ business accounts and a credit-card account.

Bellis kept digging. He saw the news articles: friends of Gibson's were speaking out; doctors were trashing her tale; there were admissions her publishers had failed to fact-check her story; sales of her book were being suspended, and then her book was being pulped; overseas book deals were being cancelled, and then her app was pulled from the Apple store. Bellis bought a copy of the May edition of the *Australian Women's Weekly*. It had Gibson's picture on the glossy front cover. He read the article, and made photocopies of the relevant pages. After Gibson went on *60 Minutes*, Hayden wrote to Channel Nine and requested the interview transcript.

It was a walk-up start. Everywhere Hayden Bellis looked, there was evidence of her claims of cancer and the conventional treatments she had never had. So, too, were there promotions for the numerous fundraising drives to raise thousands of dollars in charity money that was never passed on. Gibson's false claims were spelled out in her book, on her app descriptions, in her magazine interview, on *60 Minutes*. And, as her empire crumbled and Gibson scrubbed her lies from the internet, Bellis had little trouble recovering them: he found on Facebook a tranche of screenshots of Gibson's since-deleted posts.

Bellis served Gibson's lawyers with a notice requiring her to produce documents relating to her business activities and medical history. Later, Peter Tziotis sent another one, this time requiring Gibson to come into Consumer Affairs for questioning. She never showed. Gibson's lawyers wrote back to say Gibson had mental-health issues that could be exacerbated if she had to attend in person. Consumer Affairs issued a list of questions in writing instead.

Two months later, on Friday 6 May 2016, a text message was sent out to journalists and newsroom editors about a 12.00 pm press conference to be held that day: 'Minister Garrett to doorstop on Belle Gibson. Media Room, Level 2, 121 Exhibition St, Melb.' The Victorian government was going public with news that Belle Gibson would be prosecuted.

Jane Garrett was fresh to the job as minister for consumer affairs when Belle Gibson became a national news story. It was March

2015, and Garrett had just been sworn in to the newly elected Labor state government after spending her first four years in politics on the opposition benches. Before entering politics, Garrett was an industrial-relations lawyer who had a reputation for fighting for the underdog. She specialised in discrimination cases, and fought for causes such as women's rights at work. She's passionate about consumer rights, pursuing negligence, and defending people who have been exploited. Garrett is a straight-talker in her mid-40s, and a fierce believer in the Australian Labor Party and the trade union movement. Hanging on a wall in her home is a photo of Gough Whitlam on an iconic orange campaign poster for the Labor Party, which reads, 'It's time.' Garrett's husband, James, is a lawyer, too. They have three children and live in Carlton, in inner-city Melbourne.

When Garrett scanned the first news stories about Belle Gibson, something immediately struck a nerve. 'There is no lower form of conduct' is how she recounts her first thoughts on the scandal, over lunch at her local pub, two years later. 'I just remember being horrified by it. Disgusted by it. And then it kind of just kept getting worse and worse.' As the minister with the consumer affairs portfolio, Garrett had a front-row seat to the most appalling examples of abuse of people's fear and goodwill. She was briefed on sophisticated scams targeting the sick, the elderly, the lonely, the vulnerable. After just weeks in office, she had come to the conclusion that the only limit to evil was the human imagination. 'It's very confronting, but, of course, there's nothing worse than when it's about people's health,' Garrett says. 'You know, "scam", I think, is too light a word for this. The sense that people could be preyed on in desperate circumstances. It really is striking at the heart of human decency.'

Consumer Affairs Victoria sits within the Department of Justice, and oversees registers for operations such as funeral parlours, estate agents, car yards, and fundraisers. It handles disputes between traders and customers, and tenants and landlords, and carries out inspections, and issues product recalls. Each year, it prosecutes a few dozen cases. And, each year, it puts out a few warnings: Valentine's Day scammers targeting singles searching for love; travelling con men offering cheap repairs on roofs and driveways; small batteries that toddlers can choke on. Consumer Affairs does not have a reputation as the most proactive watchdog agency. It's seen more as a toothless tiger.

When Gibson's scam hit the headlines, there there had been a change of guard at Consumer Affairs Victoria. The agency's long-time director had just been replaced. Garrett asked her staff to schedule a meeting for her with the new appointee, a softly spoken man by the name of Simon Cohen. When she sat down with him, Garrett wanted to know what powers the government had to deal with this conduct. She made her views very clear. She told Cohen that her office took the allegations against Gibson seriously, and she demanded to know what was going to be done about it. Garrett expected Belle Gibson to be the No. 1 priority for the agency. It was a case that was close to Garrett's heart. Her mother had died from cancer in 2009. And later, in October 2016, a few months after the government sent out the media alert about her press conference, Garrett herself would be diagnosed with breast cancer. She ended up becoming the very person that she wanted to protect from Belle Gibson.

'I wasn't running down any burrow,' Garrett says, 'but I understand that feeling. It's a terrifying experience, and it can also be quite an isolating experience. And, of course, I am a person who has got means. I live, literally, under some of the best medical facilities in the world, I have access to great care, I have a voice if I want to be heard. For many, many people, cancer is a terrifying experience that is made all the worse if you're in a vulnerable state. If you're looking for comfort, or answers, or help, or salvation, or a cure, people are just ripe for this kind of exploitation. And it's just heinous, absolutely heinous, that people would do that.

'And clearly they do, and Belle is the face of it.'

From the outside, the consumer watchdog's investigation into Gibson was glacially slow; it took more than a year from the revelations that she stole fundraising dollars and lied about cancer before charges were brought against her. But within the government, Garrett was receiving weekly — sometimes daily — briefings about the case. The prosecution of Belle Gibson would become Consumer Affairs Victoria's most high-profile case in years.

The second-floor media room was packed. Journalists from the city's two daily newspapers and camera crews from every network were there. Jane Garrett and Simon Cohen arrived together, about 10 minutes late. The minister was first to take the podium. The cameras flashed. She cleared her throat.

'Ms Gibson,' she began, 'made claims some time ago that she suffered a terminal illness, a cancer, and had undertaken a course of alternative remedies and developed her own diet, which led to extreme benefits in healing. These claims were published … and have been the subject of significant controversy ever since.

'Consumer Affairs has filed in the Federal Court its first step in legal proceedings. We will be seeking substantial penalties … to ensure that [this] conduct is not undertaken again by Ms Gibson and any of the companies she may be associated with.'

The minister hit on the fact that this was a big deal; a landmark case in an age of social media. She used powerful language, and alluded to Gibson as a dangerous con artist. 'Selling people snake oil is as old as the hills,' she said, 'but its devastating damage is as fresh today. You will never put people back into the position they were in if they believed this material and this book ... but this is an important step forward.' She said it seemed Gibson thought she could get away 'scot-free'. She assured the public this would not be the case.

Before announcing the trial against Gibson, the government had already beefed up the powers of the state's health complaints watchdog so it could investigate dubious conduct by people purporting to provide health and wellness services. When debating the bill in parliament, several MPs singled out Belle Gibson as an example of the type of person operating online who could be investigated if the law was passed. Had such reforms been introduced earlier, one said, people 'might have been saved from the harm of rogue practitioners and people like Belle Gibson'. The new laws broadened the definition of what constituted a 'health service provider' to include anyone claiming to 'assess, predict, maintain or improve' a person's health. That means wellness bloggers could, for the first time, be the subject of investigation, along with dodgy medical providers and unregistered practitioners. The commissioner was also given the power to launch its own investigations (without a complaint from a victim), and could name and shame people in breach of the law by issuing public warnings. 'Under this code, no one should be making claims to cure cancer or other terminal illnesses,' commissioner Karen Cusack announced.

It's somewhat unusual to host a press conference to announce the launch of legal action like this. If anything is announced at all, it usually comes in the form of a succinct and carefully worded press release. But there was extraordinary public interest in the Belle Gibson saga, and it was an opportunity for the government to shine a spotlight on the kind of conduct she engaged in. Cancer scams are insidious, and often fly under the radar, lurking in the darkest shadows of the internet, ready to draw in those who seek them out. Now there was a face to this kind of cruelty. So, too, was it an easy opportunity for some guaranteed good press. Indeed, overall, the coverage of the announcement was extremely favourable: the minister looked tough; the government appeared principled.

An aspect of the press conference that was largely overshadowed in the summaries in TV reports and the next day's newspapers, however, was one crucial begged question. Why was Gibson being prosecuted for a civil offence, and not being charged with criminal fraud? A veteran political reporter with News Corp, who came to the press conference for a different reason — to hammer the minister about a union dispute she was involved in at the time — went on the attack. His question was straightforward. Surely this was an open-and-shut case of criminal fraud?

'Consumer Affairs and their legal team,' the minister responded, 'have explored this thoroughly and extensively. The view of the experts is that this is the best way ... my advice is this is the correct course of action.'

Consumer Affair's lawyers had met with police, and it was decided early on, within days, that police would not take action against Gibson. The Australian Competition and Consumer Commission, which runs the Scamwatch website, was also not pursuing her. Criminal charges *could* have been laid, but it's understood authorities favoured civil charges because that meant it could also hold Gibson's publisher to account. Consumer Affairs considers gaining industry-wide change to be a bigger win than claiming the scalp of one rogue operator. It was a two birds–one stone scenario: Gibson would be charged, and a warning shot would be fired across the bows of the publishing industry. The message to book publishers would be clear: you cannot absolve yourself of responsibility if you publish bullshit.

The potential civil penalties for these consumer-law breaches were no doubt hefty — up to $1.1 million for companies, and $220,000 for individuals. But Gibson's company, by this stage, was already in liquidation. The Whole Pantry was in the red, and it had a tax-office bill that needed to be settled. Gibson had no assets. And there was next to no prospect of recouping any money from her.

The action went ahead anyway. Peter Tziotis filed the writ in the Federal Court of Australia on 27 May. The first respondent was Gibson. The second was her company, Inkerman Road Nominees, which traded as The Whole Pantry (Gibson, by now, had changed the name of the business from Belle Gibson Pty Ltd). Consumer Affairs appointed a barrister named Catherine Button to argue the case on its behalf.

On Friday, 10 June 2016, Button walked through the revolving door at the corner of William Street and Latrobe Street, into the Federal Court, and into courtroom 8B for an administrative hearing. Neither Belle Gibson nor a representative of hers was anywhere to be seen. 'These are serious allegations,' Justice Mortimer said, 'and I want to make sure Ms Gibson knows the consequences of not contributing to this case.' Later, the court heard that Gibson had sent a letter to the judge's chambers 'expressly stating' that she would not be participating in the proceedings. And so the trial started without her.

Button stood up. 'By way of general background,' she began, 'Ms Gibson rose to prominence in 2013 with the launch of her app, which I assume your honour is familiar with, app being short, an abbreviation for application …'

'I even know how to use some of them, Ms Button,' Justice Mortimer replied, with a half-smile, 'so that's all right.'

'Thank you, your honour — one doesn't like to assume.'

Button carried on. 'And the app was very successful. It won

numerous prizes, it garnered Ms Gibson a very high social-media presence, and also widespread reporting on her and the success of her app in print news and online articles and the like.' The success of the app, she said, had led Gibson to a book deal. And both the app and the book were marketed and based on claims to the effect that the author had terminal cancer and had undergone conventional treatment, but had rejected them, 'in favour of a quest to heal herself naturally'.

Button told Justice Mortimer that Consumer Affairs was not accusing Gibson of explicitly saying that following her advice would cure someone's cancer. Rather, her claims of overcoming her deadly diagnosis *formed the backbone* of her media business and the context in which her products were sold. The three core claims were: (1) that she was diagnosed with terminal brain cancer in 2009; (2) that she was given four months to live; and (3) that she had taken, and then rejected, conventional medicine in favour of embarking on a quest to heal herself naturally.

There were two parts to the case, Button said: one that concerned her health claims, and the other that concerned her charitable-giving claims. Both, according to Consumer Affairs Victoria, constituted the offence of misleading and deceptive conduct.

Gibson's choice not to participate in her own trial came at a cost. Certainly, Consumer Affairs still had to carry the burden of proving its allegations on the balance of probabilities. But without any submissions by Gibson or any legal representative acting for her, she had no power to contest any of the evidence or any of the material filed against her. 'Non-participation,' warned Justice Mortimer, 'may mean that there is an absence of evidence … capable of affecting the court's evaluation.' In Gibson's absence, the trial was short. There was no need for more than one day of hearings. Button filed all of the evidence, and she said her piece. Justice Mortimer thanked her, and adjourned the case. It would be another nine months before the ruling was handed down.

A few days before the case was due back in court, Gibson appeared online again. It had been two years since she had posted anything about nutrition or given health advice online. The app was gone, her website domain had expired, and she'd closed down the @healing_belle Instagram account. But then, seemingly out of nowhere, and using her long-time pseudonym, Harry Gibson, she logged onto Facebook and went to the page of the Master Fast System, an obscure diet that espouses new-age fasting and cleansing. The diet claims it helps people 'without hope' who 'have been given a death sentence'. *Let us teach you that EVERYTHING IS POSSIBLE and your situation CAN be turned around no matter what 'they' named your disease*, its website says. The Master Fast System promotes a combination of fasting techniques, special teas, and herbs.

Gibson typed out a long and glowing review about the fad diet, and posted it to Facebook. She said she had been on the diet for just 10 days, and that already it had changed her eye colour, healed tooth cavities, and shrunk her tonsils. She went into great detail about her bowel movements, writing that she expelled a parasite and passed 'a huge rope worm', which she estimated was 60 cm long. 'I felt such HUGE relief and was floating all day afterwards.' Gibson wrote that the cure-all diet 'saved my life' and showed her 'what happiness and health looks and feels like. I feel so blessed. Thank you.' The media picked up the story, and the post was promptly removed. Gibson then shut down her personal Facebook page.

Wellness fraudster Belle Gibson is back spruiking new health advice as she prepares to face court today over false cancer claims.

Gibson was again making news on every radio station:

Disgraced blogger Belle Gibson will find out if she'll be slapped with a $1 million fine and have to offer up a public sorry for lying about having cancer. We'll be keeping you right across this one.

The nine o'clock update … Cancer con artist Belle Gibson is due to face the music in court today, with a Federal Court judge handing down a decision in a million-dollar lawsuit brought by Consumer Affairs Victoria.

It was a Tuesday in March 2017. The crews were there before the sun came up, lingering in white four-wheel drives parked along the sides of Gibson's street. They lay in wait within their cars' dim interior lights until just after dawn, when the sky lightened with shades of pink and yellow. Then, one by one, reporters in knee-length pencil skirts and in bold-coloured waistcoats emerged from the cars and made their way to the house — their cameramen, gear over shoulders, in tow. They congregated on the footpath behind Gibson's silver car, which was parked in her driveway. Neighbours returning home from early-morning swims or getting the kids out the front door for school, stared, as they always did, at the strange spectacle of a media pack in the middle of their quiet, suburban street so early in the morning. The TV crews waited, hour after hour, for Gibson to show. Every now and then, a reporter would walk up to her front door and knock. But she never came out.

Meanwhile, across town, where Peter Tziotis was waiting patiently, the clock struck 10.15 am. 'Call the first matter for judgement, please,' Justice Debbie Mortimer said, taking her seat at the bench.

'Case number VID 535-2016,' her tipstaff announced. '*The Director of Consumer Affairs Victoria and Annabelle Natalie Gibson.*'

'I have found the director has proven most but not all of the contraventions of the federal and Victorian consumer laws alleged,' Justice Mortimer said.

Belle Gibson, aged 25 years, was guilty of misleading and deceptive conduct. It was ruled that she had 'no reasonable basis' to believe she had cancer when she was making public claims about it to sell her book and her apps. And, after her general practitioner confirmed to her in November 2014 that she did not have cancer, Gibson failed to inform Apple, Google, or Penguin. Justice Mortimer found that Gibson's continued claims after this time were 'obviously false', while her claims all along that she had tried and ditched conventional treatment — the very premise of her book — were also false.

'Part of being convinced to buy what Ms Gibson was selling would involve accepting that she was not a hypochondriac or an irrational person,' the judge said, 'but an "ordinary" young woman who had suffered a tragic health event in her early life, who had nevertheless found a way to survive that event, and live with it.'

On the allegations of charity fraud, Justice Mortimer found Gibson had made deceptive and misleading representations about giving donations, and said she had 'deliberately played' the Australian public. 'Her "pitch" overwhelmingly used groups likely to evoke sympathy because of their vulnerabilities,' she said. 'Young girls, asylum seekers, sick children. Ms Gibson deliberately played on the genuine desire of members of the Australian community to help those less fortunate.'

But Justice Mortimer said she was not persuaded by Consumer Affairs' case that Gibson acted *unconscionably*. Unconscionable conduct, in Australia, is a concept that has been developed largely on a case-by-case basis. It is generally understood to mean conduct that is not just wrong or unfair, but so severe that it goes against good conscience as judged against the norms of a society. Justice Mortimer said there was not enough evidence before the court to persuade her that Gibson never *believed* her story from the outset. 'It seems to be that, at least in some respects, it might be open to find that Ms Gibson suffered from a series of delusions about her health conditions,' the judge said. 'I am not satisfied on the balance of probabilities that … Ms Gibson did not really believe she had cancer.'

The ruling was handed down, but the financial penalties against Gibson, which could be up to $1.1 million, would not be decided for another five months.

That night, Gibson logged onto Snapchat and typed out a three-word message. 'Tonight I pray.' Then the words disappeared.

Before the penalty was handed down, Justice Mortimer made a court order. She prohibited Gibson from making any more claims in connection with the sale or promotion of health and wellbeing advice about being diagnosed with brain cancer and about rejecting conventional medicine and embarking on a quest to heal herself naturally. Gibson was also ordered to pay $30,000 towards Consumer Affairs' legal costs.

On a Thursday afternoon in April 2017, a process-server from the Federal Court knocked on Gibson's front door. Clive answered. When he was asked, he gave only his first name. He would not say what his relationship with Gibson was. All he would say was that she was away and would be back in two or three weeks.

Three weeks later, on a cool Tuesday evening in May, the server returned and knocked on the door again. A young woman answered. He handed her a copy of the court's ruling, and then he asked for her full name.

'Annabelle Natalie Gibson,' she replied.

'Are you the person referred to as the first respondent in these proceedings?'

'Yes.'

Gibson closed the door and went back inside.

If Gibson read the documents she was given, she would know that if she disobeyed the order she would be 'liable to imprisonment, sequestration of property or punishment for contempt'.

Weeks went by. And then months. One of the only times Gibson made contact with the Federal Court, during its lengthy inquiry into the extent of her fraudulence, was in the last week of September 2017. It was in the form of an email — a very short one — after Justice Mortimer's assistant had written to her to advise that the penalty was about to be handed down. 'Thank you for the update,' Gibson wrote back. 'Confirming receipt of your email. Much appreciated. Belle.' Three days later, the court reconvened without her, and Justice Mortimer handed down the penalty. Belle Gibson was fined $410,000.

Justice Mortimer explained that the fine was made up of two penalties of $90,000 for Gibson's app sales and company donation claims; a $50,000 fine for her app launch donation claims; a $30,000 fine for claims about her Mother's Day fundraiser; and a $150,000 fine for her claims of donating to the family of Joshua Schwarz. The Schwarz family donation claims, Justice Mortimer said in her judgement, were the 'most serious' of Gibson's breaches. She emphasised that Gibson sought to use the family's tragedy — Joshua's terminal brain cancer diagnosis — 'for her own selfish purposes'.

'It encouraged members of the public to buy The Whole Pantry app because Ms Gibson represented she and her company would be donating 100 % of app sales that week to the Schwarz family to help Joshua Schwarz, a little boy who had an inoperable brain tumour.

In this representation, Ms Gibson expressly compared the terrible circumstances of young Joshua to her own, asserting she had the same kind of tumour as he did; a statement which was completely false. She did this to encourage members of the public to buy her product, to generate income for herself and her company, and generally to promote herself and her commercial activities. She consciously chose to use the terminal illness of a little boy in this way.'

'If ever there is conduct deserving of the label unconscionable, it is Ms Gibson's conduct in respect of Joshua.'

In setting the penalty, Justice Mortimer said there could be 'no allowance made for contrition, remorse, apology or acceptance of responsibility,' by Gibson. 'Ms Gibson had an opportunity to acknowledge her wrongdoing in the context of this proceeding,' Justice Mortimer said. 'She chose not to do so. She has chosen not to explain her conduct. She has chosen not to apologise for it.'

'Once again, it appears she has put her own interests before those of anyone else. If there is one theme or pattern which emerges through her conduct, it is her relentless obsession with herself and what best serves her interests.'

Liquidator Richard Cauchi, of insolvency firm SV Partners, said there had been 'precious little if anything' left in Gibson's company when he was appointed to wind it up in April 2016. 'There were a number of creditors, but no pot of gold,' he said. 'Consumer Affairs has obviously chosen to push as hard as it can. They understand that there is nothing to financially gain by getting an order against this company. But they want it.'

The former consumer affairs minister, Jane Garrett, when asked if she believed that any punishment under civil law could fit the crimes committed by Belle Gibson, said, 'I think we'll get to the point as a community where people like her will go to jail. Clearly, we're not there yet.'

23

KATE THOMAS — PART II

On a rainy Friday afternoon, Kate Thomas finishes her coffee at the Tall Timber café in Prahran and packs up her shiny red-and-white polka-dot bag: her 'hospital bag'. Coming here for a soy latte before appointments at The Alfred has become something of a ritual. Today's check-up is with a new oncologist, the fifth she's had at the hospital in less than two years. Just before 1.30 pm, Kate gathers her things and zips up her matching polka-dot raincoat. And, like she's done dozens of times before, she walks down busy Commercial Road.

The oncology waiting room is drab. On its walls are pictures of flowers and landscapes and information posters about public-health services. It's what she calls the 'smell of sickness' that Kate dreads most about this room. She hates it here. Most of the time, she comes by herself. 'I didn't want anyone else to feel that sickness,' she said. Kate takes out a pale-green expanding file from her hospital bag, and starts thumbing through the folders and sleeves inside. Scripts. Pathology results. IVF information. Radiation.

Chemo. Surgery.

Kate stands out from the other patients in the room. They are all older than her, and they all look sicker. There's an elderly man wearing a yellow-and-white cap, slumped low in the back of a chair. A woman in a black beanie sits alone, watching a daytime soap on the TV perched in the top corner of the room. A man with a drawn face sits in silence, leafing through a magazine. A skinny Asian man comes and goes from the room. A gaunt-looking woman in maroon glasses sits in a wheelchair next to a man, presumably her husband, who's reading the newspaper. He tries to help her take off her cardigan, but stops when they squabble about which sleeve to tackle first. A mother and her middle-aged adult daughter sit side by side, staring down at the iPhones in their laps. The older woman raises hers to her chin and whispers orders, trying to work Siri.

It's time to go in. The consultation room is just a desk, a couple of chairs, a sink, and an examination bed. The window looks out to the brick wall of one of the hospital's other wings. Rain belts against the glass. Dr Maggie Moore asks Kate how she's doing. They talk about osteoporosis — whether or not she definitely has it. Judging by recent bone-density scans, the doctor fears she might. And they discuss changing one of her medicines in the hope it might lift her chance of survival, or at the least improve her quality of life. They talk about putting her onto a new medicine — six doses, every six months. 'I want to maximise my chances,' Kate tells her new doctor.

It's during this consultation that Kate learns more bad news. The cancer she has — invasive ductal carcinoma NST (of no specific type) — is even more serious than suspected. The diagnosis was grade three, stage 3b. Dr Moore looks over her papers. It's actually stage 3c, the most serious type before stage 4 — terminal. Kate looks like she's been winded.

'That's the first time I've heard "c",' she says. Her shoulders and head drop, but she quickly tries to pick herself up. 'That's OK. That's alright. It is what it is. Yep, I'd still rather know.'

Kate and Nik live in the salt-sprayed suburb of St Kilda West, a short stroll down the beach from the loft that Gibson lived in at the height of her fame. Her ground-floor art-deco apartment is spotless, and stylishly decorated with mid-century furniture. Everything looks like it has its place.

During her treatment, Kate kept working. She was the manager of a café called Cornerstone & Co, south-east of Melbourne, past Gibson's townhouse, in the vibrant bayside suburb of Hampton. A regular patron, Gibson used to go to the café with her son, Oli, then a toddler, and her partner, Clive. Kate got comfort from seeing her idol in the flesh. She admired her. 'She always looked so healthy. I always thought, *How can you look so good when your cancer's probably way worse than mine, and yet I've got no hair, no eyebrows, no eyelashes, I've got sunken eyes, I'm bloated?* I just looked horrendous,' she said.

A year into her treatment, in early March 2015, Kate read about Gibson's scam when it made headlines: *Friends and doctors raise doubts over 'Healing Belle' cancer claims ... Mega-blogger Belle Gibson casts doubt on her own cancer claims ... Supporters turn on Belle Gibson as cancer claims unravel.*

Kate had just finished radiation. The news stories flashed up on her iPhone while she was on a lunch break at the café. Kate seethed. She felt betrayed, duped, taken advantage of. But she realised how lucky she was that she hadn't been sucked in all the way. Now, she worries about the other cancer sufferers who posted their solidarity with Gibson and who pledged to shun their doctors' advice.

'I saw so many people making comments about following her

and not doing conventional medicine,' Kate says, 'and I just don't know how she can live with herself. People would be saying, "You're such an inspiration, I've decided not to do chemo, I don't want to put that toxic stuff in my body, I'm just going to eat healthy and do a juicing fast-type diet." Belle would have been reading those comments and knowing that people were stopping treatment. That is not OK. People are vulnerable — you would do anything to survive longer or to not have to deal with that horrible toxic stuff going through your body.'

Kate ripped Gibson's book to shreds, scrunched it up, and set it on fire. She wanted to hurt Gibson by torturing the book. She burnt it, one page at a time, until it was black. 'I didn't want it to just go up in flames,' she said. 'She didn't deserve flames.'

As though it were yesterday, Kate remembers the first time she saw Gibson back at the café after everything had come out. It was on the weekend, and the place was heaving with customers. Kate watched Gibson enter with her son and a man, sit silently, and look over the menu. Kate wanted to say something, yell something, but she didn't want to make a scene. So she didn't. But she drew the line at waiting on her.

'Kate was quite shaken,' recalled her boss, Michelle Pavone. 'She felt completely let down … it definitely unsettled the team, because we had been supporting Kate through her journey. Everyone was a bit disturbed by her presence.'

Gibson came in a couple more times when Kate was working. Each time, Kate would drop whatever she was doing at the time and walk out of the building. She would never serve her. 'I would always look her in the eye, but I couldn't say anything,' she said. 'I was so angry.'

'It's just that I was invested for so long, and I've been through hell and back, and she's just living her life. Even what she's going through now is absolutely nothing compared to what people fighting cancer go through. I have to work, but my body is failing me, and this witch of a person is still unaffected by all the lies she told and all the sick people she preyed on.

'I don't even hate cancer, but I hate her.'

When you're in your early 30s, things start to change, and they start changing pretty quickly: friends get engaged and get married; people buy houses; some become pregnant and soon start families. Kate and Nik were on par with their friends, until the cancer put their lives on a completely different course.

'We just sort of stopped,' Kate says. 'And I would feel like such a downer being around my friends when they have all these happy things happening in their lives. They are all moving forward, which is great … but it's been hard for me to watch and be around.'

'It's an isolating experience,' adds Nik. 'People said afterwards they didn't know what to say. But nothing, silence, is the worst thing. It makes you feel even more alone.'

Kate's intense medication has put her into menopause, meaning there is no way she will be able to have a baby. She and Nik were not planning on having children soon, but in a few years they would probably have been ready. They had both talked about it before, and saw it in their future — once they had a bit more financial security and a house of their own. 'That choice is taken away,' Kate says.

(chewed)

The skin around Kate's nails is red-raw. Her foot bounces off the waiting-room floor. It's 10 days since the doctor found a suspect lump where her left breast used to be. It was not there at her check-up a month earlier. Today, Kate will have an ultrasound over the reconstruction. The hope is that this will rule out secondary cancer. It is almost 3.00 pm on a Tuesday in the middle of summer, and next month marks three years since the cancer was found. Kate is a ball of nervous energy.

'Katherine?'

The sonographer appears from around the corridor. She is middle-aged and kind-looking, and wears her red-brown hair in a ponytail.

'Follow me, please.'

Kate stands up and reaches behind her, clamping shut the white hospital gown with her fist. She shuffles down the corridor, awkwardly holding her bags and trying to secure the piece of twill tape on the back of the gown. It is no use. Half her back is exposed; tattoos flash through the slit.

It does not really bother Kate, though. She is used to the clinical, impersonal way that she is seen by medical staff. And nothing — nothing — could be worse than the first time. It was before the reconstruction surgery. Kate was standing in front of a team of seven specialists, all men, when she was asked to remove her gown. They had to mark her body with ink. They planned to go in through her thigh, take the fat from her stomach, rebuild her breast. 'It was everything,' Kate says, 'I was just standing there naked while they marked me with the texta.'

Halfway down the corridor is Room 2 — Outpatient Ultrasound. Kate is ushered through the heavy sliding door and towards the bed in the middle of the room. The sonographer asks Kate where the lump is, when she found it, what it feels like. Kate has never touched it; the last time she found a knurled mass in her breast, everything changed.

Kate tells her the lump is at eleven o'clock, loosens the gown, and lies down on her back. When the wand presses into the red scar tissue, a black-and-white image flashes up on the monitor. It looks like a moonscape. The wand starts at the top of the scar, which is shaped like the ring left under a saucer, moving anti-clockwise.

The wand slides across the skin through sticky, cerulean gel, trawling the fat and glandular tissue and muscle beneath for something sinister. Kate looks over her right shoulder towards the monitor as the machine starts making hospital noises. *Buleep. Buleep.* The dull beeps ring out in the darkened room.

'I'm just documenting it,' the sonographer says.

'Uh-huh,' Kate replies, as she lies there tensely.

The wand stops sliding when it comes to the dip in her armpit. It lingers, moves on, comes back. Then it goes to the breastbone, then higher, to the bony plate just below the neck. It stops again. Every time it does, Kate squints in on the grainy, upside-down picture.

'I'm just pressing in sometimes to see a bit deeper,' the sonographer says.

'Uh-huh.'

The clicking starts. Each click is a photo. 'We document everything we see.'

'Uh-huh.'

A heavy silence fills the room. After a few minutes, the sonographer says she needs to see the radiologist to make sure there are enough images to figure out what the lump is. She leaves the room. Five minutes pass. Those minutes that Kate spends lying on the bed alone in the dark seem like much longer. When the radiologist, a woman, returns with the sonographer, Kate searches her face for clues. But she gives nothing away. Both specialists stand at the monitor. Kate's lips are pressed firmly together; her legs are stiff. The sonographer takes the wand, and presses into the scar tissue again. *Buleep.* A dark, oval-shaped mass bursts onto the screen.

'We can see the lump,' the radiologist says. 'It doesn't look like it's very vascular and solid, which is a good thing. It's going from the top right down to the chest wall.'

The radiologist says she thinks the growth is a cyst. She is not too worried about it, but she orders a mammogram anyway. If it is not clear from the mammogram whether the lump is suspicious, a biopsy will then need to be performed.

Kate has the mammogram, and leaves the hospital. She crosses Commercial Road, and walks into the park to find her parents, Greg and Jennie. They're walking Brando; medical appointments like these are too much for them to bear.

The next day, Kate sends a text message. 'It's a bloody two-centimetre oily cyst! Yay, a cyst. I'm on the way to work feeling relief.'

Kate's five-year goal is to be cancer-free. If she makes it to February 2019 without a recurrence or secondary cancer, she and Nik will try to have a baby. Before she started treatment, she underwent IVF, salvaging and freezing five eggs. Kate won't be able to carry a child herself anymore, but there are other options. She's positive, but realistic. Although shaken by the news that two of her dearest friends, both young mothers, were recently told their breast cancers had recurred and were terminal, Kate tries to be optimistic. 'Half the battle is just having a positive attitude to life,' Kate says. 'But that hasn't wavered for me. I want to be here, I want to have a family, I love my life. I just have to get to that first five years. And then 10.'

24

SOCIAL MEDIA VERSUS THE MEDIA

'Two things about Belle Gibson are hard to believe,' began an article in the December 2014 edition of the popular women's magazine *Elle*. 'The first is that she's only 26 years old, and the second is that she has terminal brain cancer.'

Both of these statements, it turned out, were hard to believe for a very good reason: they were not true. But in the months and years before this would be revealed, the staff at *Elle* was far from the only ones in the media who deserted journalism's chief responsibility — to report the news accurately and fairly — in their eagerness to capitalise on the remarkable Gibson and her hard-to-believe tale.

There's an old saying in the news business: 'Any story that looks too good to be true, probably is.' Yet, increasingly, this warning is routinely ignored by respected media outlets and their staff. Dubious claims and outright falsehoods are regularly being reported as facts. Stories that are wildly exaggerated or totally fabricated are being printed and published (and thereby given greater legitimacy) by professionals whose job is meant to be to distinguish truth from fiction, to debunk lies, to be a source of accurate information. Times have changed. And, as news outlets follow their audiences and advertisers into an unfamiliar world, standards have slid. The new world of news is a digital world, where the revenue needed to keep news platforms afloat is driven largely by the number of clicks stories can get. It's a world where social media is king, and 'viral' is the name of the game, and where rumours, hoaxes, and misinformation have the power to spread with unprecedented ease. News travels fast. But lies, it seems, can fan out ever faster.

Perhaps you remember, while scrolling through your social feeds some years ago, the story of a 21-year-old Florida woman who captivated the internet after claiming she'd had a third breast implanted — and the pictures to prove it. 'A woman has spent $20,000 on surgery to get a third breast,' said a news.com.au piece, widely syndicated and accompanied by a selfie-photo gallery of her triple-breasted chest:

> The Florida massage therapist, who calls herself Jasmine Tridevil, said she had the surgery a few months ago. 'It was really hard finding someone that would do it, too, because they're breaking the code of ethics,' she said. 'I called like 50 or 60 doctors, nobody wanted to do it.'

The story stemmed from an interview the woman gave on Real Radio 104.1, a local station out of Orlando, Florida. It ended up in the *New York Post*, CBS, Fox News, *The Telegraph*, and the *Daily Mail*. News sites and TV stations all over the globe ran with the story (and, of course, the attention-grabbing photos of her third breast that, it later turned out, was a wearable prosthetic).

'It was the perfect encapsulation of everything that can be wrong with viral news,' says Craig Silverman, from web giant BuzzFeed.

'This is a story that just had huge red flags from the get-go; not just huge anatomical, surgical, and physiological red flags about whether this could be even done, but the way no one made any effort to do any additional verification because it was such a "too good to check" story.'

Some articles that covered it used hedging language, such as *claims*, or used inverted commas, conveying that the information they were passing on was unverified, but they wanted to run with it anyway. It took roughly 48 hours for the story to be debunked entirely. But once it was, 'not as many news organisations covered it,' Silverman says, 'and many who had [initially] covered it as true, failed to update their stories.'

Craig Silverman is BuzzFeed Canada's media editor. His office in the city of Toronto, where, just past 5.00 pm on a summer evening, he finds a quiet room to answer our call on Skype. He's wearing a buttoned shirt and white earphones, and starts by telling us about what it is that he does. Silverman is not a typical media editor. He doesn't cover media-industry acquisitions, or hirings, or share-price fluctuations, like his counterparts at most other news companies. Instead, Silverman is pretty much exclusively focused on the upsurge of online misinformation, the emergence of deliberately 'fake news', and the way that Facebook and Twitter and other powerful social-media platforms are changing the way information flows. The way people are receiving it. The way people are consuming it. And, most importantly, how newsrooms are dealing with it. In 2014, he released a landmark research paper, *Lies, Damn Lies and Viral Content*. Published by the Tow Center at Columbia University's Journalism School, it analysed more than 1,600 news articles about more than 100 online rumours that circulated in the press over a period of several months. The findings were not good.

'It's a vicious-yet-familiar cycle,' his paper stated. 'A claim makes its way to social media or elsewhere online. One or a few news sites choose to repeat it ... Within minutes or hours, a claim can morph from a lone tweet or badly sourced report to a story repeated by dozens of news websites, generating tens of thousands of shares.'

News media have always made gaffes. And reporters have always made errors. But, Silverman contends, never quite like this; never quite so often. Today, rumours and unverified information make their way online and find an audience faster and with a degree of abundance that's 'unlike anything in the history of journalism or communication'. One of the biggest and perhaps most overlooked shifts in the news industry since the arrival of social media has been that journalists' position as the *gatekeepers* of information is now utterly eroded. Stories and individuals can shoot from obscurity to popularity without going through the checks and balances that were once provided by the traditional media. This change is not all bad, of course. The upside is that we are exposed to a greater diversity of voices and interesting viewpoints, outside the mainstream, that once may have been sidelined or muted. But the downside of all this is that, sometimes, the things that now flow through unchecked and unverified also include distortions, hoaxes, or dangerous lies, being peddled by dangerous liars.

'Usually the approach of a journalist in a newsroom has been to say, "Oh, I can't figure out if this rumour is true or false. So I won't write anything about it",' Silverman explains, 'because it wasn't something that was getting wide dissemination; it was just something they had heard as a tip. But, today, that thing might already have 10,000 retweets. It may already being going off on Facebook. And so it changes the way journalists engage with information.'

An aspiration shared by both traditional publishers and the new league of web-only news organisations is to plug into what's trending and attracting attention online. The story of the three-breasted woman was no isolated incident. Examples abound. In September 2015, the media leapt on an uploaded YouTube video of a beautiful French tourist, Natalie Amyot, who claimed she was seeking help to find an Australian man with whom she had had a one-night stand and who, she said, was the father of her unborn baby. The video attracted more than three million views, and went viral, assisted in no small part by the fact that it was picked up and embedded in online stories on news sites everywhere. It was later outed as a marketing stunt. 'Did anyone check if Natalie's remarkable story was true?' asked host Paul Barry on ABC's *Media Watch* the following week. 'Well, one or two tried, but most obeyed the modern media dictum, which is "File first, ask questions later."'

Then, just two months later, something else that began trending on social media set off another storm of online articles. It was the story of a man with a most unfortunate name. 'If you have ever thought your name sounded bad, spare a thought for this guy,' began one article from November 2015. The Vietnamese–Australian man, who said his name was Phuc Dat Bich, became a big story amid claims that Facebook's 'discriminatory' moderating systems had been repeatedly shutting his page down for having a false or misleading name. 'Apparently his name is unremarkable in Vietnam,' said an article on *New York* magazine's website, 'yet ostensibly global-minded Facebook is still giving him trouble. So he posted his passport for proof. And please, if you meet him, it's pronounced "Foo Da Bic."' Based on a doctored screenshot of a passport (shared 123,000 times) and a post he put on Facebook, the story appeared everywhere: on the BBC, Sky News, *The Guardian*, and *The Mirror*. The author, referring to himself as 'Mr. T', eventually bragged on Facebook that it was all a hoax, and made some poignant criticism of the reporters who had swallowed it whole: 'Out of this ordeal I've concluded not to trust the credibility of the media, it's twisted by the hungry journalists who mask the truth … It goes to show that an average Joe like myself can con the biggest news [organisations] with ease.'

Examining this troubling trend of the news covering unverified online content, you need look no further than what happened with Belle Gibson. Her story ticked all boxes. It was heart-warming. It made us feel good. But, most of all, it was one we *wanted* to believe: the story of the human spirit defeating a dangerous and deadly disease. And Gibson, the woman at the centre of it all, was a young mum, inspiring and photogenic. Her story appealed to emotions, not logic. It was picked up everywhere, and featured far and wide.

During their inquiries into the extent of her fraudulence, investigators from Consumer Affairs hired a well-known media-monitoring service to collate all media reports and articles, across print, broadcast, and digital, using the search parameters 'Belle Gibson' and 'The Whole Pantry', from 20 August 2013 to 6 March 2015 — the day before *The Age* exposed her unlawful fundraising appeals.

In all, there had been 550 glowing reports, including syndications, across all news platforms, with a cumulative reach of more than 13.3 million people. The cost of the advertising space, the report said, would have been more than $4.6 million. The stories were circulated in every state and territory in Australia.

The *Elle* article, a multi-page spread, was headlined, 'The Most Inspiring Woman You've Met This Year'. A feature piece in a weekend magazine began, 'Instagram is full of inspirational quotes, but few ring as true as those posted by @Healing_Belle's Belle Gibson.' A *Herald Sun* headline called her the 'Melbourne mum … taking the world by storm'.

'If anyone bragged they were a game-changer,' the article said, 'odds are you'd call them up themselves. But coming from Belle Gibson, it's pure truth.'

Everywhere, her story was recklessly recounted as fact. Belle Gibson bypassed the verification process that might have applied if she had called up a newsroom and claimed to have cured an incurable cancer with healthy eating. Her story had gained attention online — to the tune of 200,000 followers — and had stamps of approval from Penguin and Apple. For time-poor reporters and editors, often fuelled by the unrelenting pressure to 'get the story up' as quickly as possible, important questions are often pushed to one side.

On one occasion, when an editor responded to a pitch from a journalist who had interviewed Gibson, she asked for more details, but the reporter couldn't get more time with her. 'I didn't have too long with her, so I am trying to piece together what I have,' they said. 'Fascinating story — she's just been told she now has kidney cancer.' The story ran anyway.

'Media have often fallen for the hard-luck and miraculous recovery story,' says Craig Silverman, and what makes it harder is the reluctance of reporters to 'prod them, and say, "Well, can you show us a medical bill? Who's your doctor, and can I talk to them?" The right thing,' he says, 'is to have a policy in a newsroom and to say unless we have a statement from a hospital or a doctor, then we can't go and write the miraculous-recovery story. It's easy to say that after the fact, but we have to be aware of our willingness to be deceived.'

Getting information about a person's medical condition can be difficult, however, even with their consent. In the case of Monique Watt, the young woman with brain cancer from earlier in this book, it took almost nine weeks to confirm basic information with her treating doctors, even after she gave permission for them to discuss her case. Given the subject matter of this book, we wanted to clarify not only Monique's cancer diagnosis, which was detailed on medical paperwork she provided, but also her prognosis, which was not readily available to us. So we contacted the media unit at the Austin Hospital, where Monique is treated. We were given the runaround for two months. At first, we were advised that Monique's verbal consent was sufficient to discuss her case. Later, the hospital required her consent in writing. The hospital repeatedly asked for Monique's name, her phone number, and about the information we were seeking. The deputy communications manager suggested we 'bank on leaving us out of this' after there was no response from Monique's neurosurgeon to our follow-up emails. There were numerous unreturned messages. When the deputy communications manager stopped replying to emails, we contacted the director of communications, who never responded to our messages or returned phone calls.

We can only assume that The Austin's position was the same as others — that they did not want their organisation to be associated with the Belle Gibson scam. In the end, after more than 40 email exchanges and a dozen phone conversations between us, the media unit, and three neurosurgeons at the hospital, we were given the information we requested. Journalists face pressing deadlines on a daily basis, and, in an age when institutions are more tightly media-managed than ever before, they are constantly facing roadblocks that restrict access to information. What this means is that it is becoming harder and harder to verify and fact-check questionable claims.

The Belle Gibson case throws up dilemmas not just for journalists, but for any organisation planning to use social media to grow its brand. In this modern world of online influencers — people who are paid to endorse products and services, often without explicitly saying so — businesses now face a new risk: partnering with a fake. Australian media agency Mumbrella promoted a September 2017 seminar by asking, *Has Belle Gibson ruined influencers for health marketers?* The session, titled 'The Belle Gibson Factor: The Pitfalls (And Benefits) of Using Influencers in The Health Space', heard from public-relations and legal experts who discussed the challenges of using influencers and, crucially, how to spot 'a fake'.

Tim Crowe strode to the front of the room, took the microphone, and turned to face the crowd. He'd been invited to the Peter MacCallum Cancer Centre, as part of a professional-development program, to give a presentation to the hospital's dietitians. Tim had a feel for the room. He had once been a dietitian here himself, about 15 years before, working on the wards, in clinics and in chemotherapy units, providing nutrition advice to cancer patients. But the topic of his talk today was not about his career or about the past. It was about something intensely modern; something that was having a profound impact in the field of cancer care, but which most professionals still knew very little about.

Tim's talk was on social media — in particular, the dangers of social-media-driven nutrition messages, which clinical dietitians these days can no longer simply try to ignore. The opening slide flashed up the title of his presentation: *What Dietitians Need to Know in the Post-Belle Gibson World.*

'I seem to be speaking more to professionals these days about social media than I do about all the nerdy stuff I've spent my career doing,' Tim began. 'But it's something I'm very passionate about, and excited to talk about.'

Whether it is Facebook, Twitter, YouTube, Instagram, Snapchat, or blog platforms like Wordpress, Tim explains, one in seven people living in Australia and the US reports using social media. And the dawn of these new technologies has had reverberating effects across the world. They have changed the way we interact, the way we run our businesses, the way we live our lives. And, according to a survey by PriceWaterhouseCoopers, they have changed the way we look at our health. More than 75 per cent of Americans aged 18–50 use social media to research symptoms and seek out advice about medical conditions. Millennials, the survey found, were the most likely to see social media as a trusted source of health information. The phenomenon is termed the 'Dr Google effect'.

People now have more access to information than ever before, and that can be a great thing, giving patients more input in the decisions being made about diagnoses and treatment. For the first time, patients and caregivers with no medical training can become engaged in learning about their options, download journal articles, and seek out information such as clinical-trial opportunities, from outside sources. But, further, the online experience has come to entail more than just collecting information. Social-media networks have also ended up as hugely beneficial support networks, too, which let patients and caregivers share their experiences with each other and not feel so alone. 'There is an additional network they can access outside of the chemotherapy day ward,' Tim explained, 'outside of their treating physician and health professionals that allows emotional support, help and advice. It can be a wonderful thing.'

But then there are dangers, Tim tells the room. Social media permits inexpert advice to spread as widely as evidence-based information from reputable health organisations.

'Once upon a time you had to do a lot of digging to find out the truth about how to really heal cancer,' Jess Ainscough once posted to her followers. 'These days, as more and more people are fed up with conventional options, searching for something better and discovering that there is something better, they are doing everything in their power to make sure the word is spread far and wide. I thank Facebook, Twitter and the mass inundation of awesome blogs out there for this.'

According to an analysis by *The Independent*, out of the 20 most-shared articles on Facebook in 2016 with the word 'cancer' in the headline, more than half contained claims discredited by doctors and health authorities. The vast amounts of anecdotal information and unsupported claims of cures that are available online, Tim said, can confuse patients' decision-making process. For two months in 2016, readers of his website, *Thinking Nutrition*, sent him a stream of inquiries about the cancer-killing properties of crushed avocado seeds. A video had gone viral on Facebook, with more than 25 million views, claiming the seed is the most nutrient-dense part of the avocado, and demonstrating how you can prepare the seed for consumption. When it comes to social media and cancer, a lot of what dietitians today need to do revolves around 'debunking' the supposed benefits of avocado seeds, cleanses, detoxes, coffee enemas, or eating shark cartilage. 'If someone is really convinced this is the pathway for them,' Tim posited, 'how do you try to give them a bit more factual information so they don't go down the whole Belle Gibson route and expunge all therapies whatsoever?'

The extraordinary story of Belle Gibson has been a flashpoint of sorts. There are information bubbles out there in the world of social media, a world where truth and opinion are difficult to distinguish, and where the most evidence-based claims are not necessarily the most exciting ones. And they have the potential to influence vulnerable cancer patients down the dangerous path of non-evidence-based treatments.

'Why Belle and Jess [Ainscough] got the notoriety they did was because of the stories they had … of beating cancer with healthy, clean eating,' Tim said. 'That's much more powerful than talking about how there is no evidence that following a particular diet can cure cancer. That's boring!'

So, Tim asked the room of dietitians, what should they be doing about it? Find the good ones. There *are* good social-media pages out there, which are credible and well-moderated and are not going to fill cancer patients' heads full of fiction and false promises. As well, dietitians should become more active on social media, and, where possible, engage in discussions. 'If you have enough fact-checkers,' he said, 'you can stop the spread of a myth.' Last, when patients of theirs say they want to try a fad diet they've been reading about on social media, resist the urge to tell them they are wrong. Focus on the positives first, such as the fact that the diet does encourage more real foods and less junk. Listen carefully to their position, why they have done what they've done, and give them options, rather than telling them what to do. 'Nudging,' Tim said, 'that's the big word in health promotion.'

In a 2015 article in the *Medical Journal of Australia*, Melbourne oncologist Ian Haines wrote about the changing way in which patients seek out information about alternative cancer therapies. Ian started working in this field in the early 1980s. He said there have always been people claiming to cure their cancer with diet, but where that was once confined to the self-help sections of bookstores, patients are now constantly being 'beckoned, assailed and seduced' online.

'More of these claims appear to be coming from individuals with implausible claims of advanced cancer and "self cure",' Ian said, citing the example of the ex-model who promoted the pineapple cure. 'Some of these claims are wrapped in a cloak of pseudo-scientific tests and research to give them greater credibility.'

Ian and his colleagues continue to see patients opting for extreme dietary and alternative treatments for potentially curable cancers. He said these patients often don't return to conventional medicine until the cancer has spread and become incurable. 'To see patients with early disease, who would have an excellent prognosis if standard treatment protocols were followed, return with advanced disease after eschewing this standard treatment for dietary cures, is extremely distressing for the patients, their loved ones and their treating doctors,' he wrote.

In 30 years, Ian said, he has never seen a patient who pursued a purely dietary treatment and whose progress exceeded the expectations for their particular cancer.

25

LIFE AFTER BELLE GIBSON

In the story room at the RTÉ headquarters in south Dublin, a group of writers is trying to get inside the head of a compulsive liar. They're huddled around a laptop with cups of tea and canteen chocolate bars, transfixed by what they're watching on the small screen. Every now and then they look at each other, mouths agape. This is the writing team behind Ireland's longest-running soap opera, *Fair City*. It's late 2016, and they're about to bring an old character back to the show — Heather, a successful novelist with a dark side. She suffers from Munchausen by proxy syndrome, and will go on to poison her 12-year-old daughter to garner sympathy and love from her family and friends. These writers need to understand what drives a serial manipulator. They need to make her human. Believable.

Belle Gibson's *60 Minutes* interview has become compulsory viewing for anyone on the show who comes into contact with Heather's character. 'By nature of Munchausen by proxy syndrome, the abuser will often never admit or even believe they were in the wrong,' series consultant Sam Atwell says. 'We needed to find a real-life counterpart, who, on the surface, appeared to be absolutely genuine and with everyone's best interest at heart, whilst also being capable of horrendously destructive acts.' Atwell, an Australian, was an actor and then a director on *Home and Away*. He left Sydney in 2014, and landed the job in Ireland as script producer on *Fair City* soon after. He's been captivated by Gibson's story ever since it broke.

On a rainy Tuesday afternoon, about a year after Gibson admitted to lying, and 17,000 kilometres from Melbourne, Atwell sent an email out to his team of 50 researchers, writers, and editors. 'I think we are looking for something deeper and a little scarier for Heather's return,' he began. Atwell then introduced the young Australian woman who told the world she was curing herself of terminal brain cancer without medicine. He attached the televised interview. This, he told his team, was the 'benchmark' for Heather. The response from the writers was unanimous. The footage was disturbing, they agreed, and perfect inspiration for their character. 'I think Heather being all about love and healing is great,' one replied. 'Belle Gibson talks all the time about love and respect and also how SHE is the victim. She's also very articulate and fearless! And Heather is all these things too.'

Atwell says using Gibson as a real-life case study helped the writers present Heather as a character who was 'constantly teetering on the edge of madness'. Ultimately, he says, the Gibson case was a catalyst for powerful, divisive drama. 'Just as with the story of Belle Gibson, we wanted to portray a character that compelled our audience to battle between being intrigued, almost feeling sorry for her, but then wanting to scream at the television for our other characters to wake up to Heather's nefarious motives and actions,' he says. 'Indeed, it feels like the stuff that soap-opera writers dream up.'

***

Belle Gibson lives with her partner, Clive, and son, Oli, in an Edwardian joined house in the inner-city suburb of Northcote, a multicultural neighbourhood in Melbourne's north. Their single-storey home sits behind a white picket fence and large, flowering white rose shrubs. Gibson's silver Subaru Forester is parked in the driveway. In the mornings, Clive walks his stepson to the local station, where they catch the train together to Oli's school. Last year, Clive took Oli to one of their neighbour's Christmas parties. Gibson didn't go. She keeps a low profile. The neighbours know who she is, but most have never spoken to her. 'Sometimes she'll wave, but that's it,' said one. 'It's all very strange,' said another.

Gibson looks different now from how she once appeared in public. She fashioned herself as a good-food guru, someone who lived and breathed the wellness message; but, after everything came crashing down, that persona melted away. These days, she looks like she's trying to blend into the crowd. Designer dresses have been replaced with dark-coloured tights and hoodies. The Instagram account that catapulted her to success is gone. So is her old Facebook account.

When former friends see Gibson in the street, they turn around and walk the other way. People are always surprised when they catch a glimpse of her eating dinner on Lygon Street, or having drinks at Cookie in the city, or skiing in the Victorian alps. 'She goes about her business,' said one. 'She goes out with Clive, gallivanting around like nothing happened.' We spoke to only one person from Gibson's old life, a Melbourne business owner, who said they had stayed in contact with her. 'I don't agree with what she's done, and I'm ashamed that she's done it, but it's not my place to judge her,' they said. 'She needs support, and she needs a friend.'

The people who were swept up in Gibson's world, the people who worked alongside her, are less forgiving. 'She has no remorse,' said someone with whom she worked with closely. 'No remorse for her actions or the harm she has caused. She never apologised for anything, publicly or personally. I just want it behind me, and everyone who worked on her book and app is in the same mindset; they just want to let it go. We don't need it to be replayed to us. She destroyed people's careers at Apple and Penguin. I'm just glad the truth has come out.'

And then there are the fans, some of whom have been unable to reconcile her deception. For some cancer sufferers and their families, Gibson will always be a lightning rod for their anger. One patient, Australian author Julia Watson, wrote about Belle Gibson on her blog in April 2015. It was re-published by Fairfax Media under the headline, 'Why I will never forgive Belle Gibson.' Julia, a mother-of-four, had bowel cancer, and died in late 2016. This post has been reproduced with permission from her husband, Gary:

> December 11, 2013 was a golden day. I remember it well; how sunny it was, the light that shone through the window and lit up my children's hair as I looked at them in the rearview mirror. I told them we would take them to the beach that night, and we talked about how much we were looking forward to Santa, and our annual Christmas holidays. It was a day so filled with promise. It was, in fact, a LIFE filled with promise.
>
> We never went to the beach that night. Instead, the children marked their afternoon being minded by the staff in an endoscopy clinic while a doctor showed my husband and me a photo of a large, obstructive, and he assured us, definitely malignant tumour in my bowel. Further scans showed that it had jumped ship to my liver and the fight was almost certainly going to be unwinnable.
>
> And just like that, I would never know another golden day.
>
> A week later, I left the oncologists office with a plan – and a booking at the local chemotherapy unit. While calm in manner,

and kind, he pulled no punches. We were talking about very advanced cancer, and if I didn't respond to chemotherapy, my life expectancy would be measured in mere months, perhaps no more than three. Even with a good response, we were likely to be only talking about a year or two.

As someone with a genuine phobia of vomiting, I was scared all my life that one day I would get cancer and have to have chemotherapy. Pure poison, it might give me a little longer in the lives of my children and those who love me, but would surely make me hairless, haunted looking, and way too familiar with what the bottom of the toilet bowl looked like. I'll be honest and say I wasn't sure I could do it, but I looked at my four beautiful daughters, and the devastated face of the man who thought he would grow old with me by his side, and knew that do it I must.

It's not hard for me to imagine how it could have gone another way. I could have come home that day, and a quick Google search on 'how to cure your own cancer' would have taken me to the blogs and websites of 'wellness warriors' like Belle Gibson and Jess Ainscough. I could have pored over the stories of these 'inspirational women' for hours, both with diagnoses of terminal cancer, but none of the grey eyes, sallow skin, and carefully drawn-on eyebrows. These women GLOWED with vitality and health; their hair, all natural, shone. Their eyes twinkled.

In the desperate hours and weeks after I was diagnosed, while I came to terms with the imminent end of my life, it would have been so easy for me to believe that if these women cured themselves on a diet of whole food, kilos of vegetable juices a day, and a few litres of coffee up the clacker, so could I. Maybe I didn't have to have a plastic disc parked in my chest to deliver the poison. Maybe I didn't have to wake up to a pillow covered in hair. Best of all, maybe I didn't have to DIE.

It may be hard to believe that anyone could be that naive. But let me tell you, there is nothing more compelling than a glimmer of hope offered by women with unlined hands and healthy nails, and seemingly the potential for long and healthy lives. Woman who were once JUST LIKE YOU, pregnant with deadly malignancies, cured without one single bag of cytotoxic chemicals delivered into their bloodstream.

I didn't seek an 'alternative' path to cure my cancer, opting for what has been a brutal but proven protocol to extend my life. Because chemotherapy has 'worked' for me, I have had 15 months of precious time, time that has allowed me to experience and enjoy and watch my children grow, and the potential is still there for much more time.

2015 has been a spectacularly bad year for the 'wellness warrior'. Jess Ainscough, who did have cancer, and opted to treat herself with the controversial Gerson therapy, is dead. Jess' mother, who eschewed the conventional medicine that could have possibly saved her life, in order to follow her daughter into alternative therapies to cure her breast cancer, has also been dead for two years. Every bit as dead as I would be if I had not reported to that chemotherapy ward at three-weekly intervals.

And what of Belle Gibson? Well, Belle is not dead, because she was never dying. Her terminal brain cancer that she had 'cured' herself of was simply a figment of her imagination. The lucrative wellness industry, born out of this lie, now lies in tatters. Also in tatters are the lives, hopes and dreams of Christ knows how many desperate souls who hung onto every word she said.

And that alone is the reason I can't forgive Belle Gibson. She would like us to see her as a victim — that a difficult childhood robbed her of her relationship with the truth, and indeed reality. I like to think of myself as a compassionate person, and I can feel a little bit for her there. Yep, she f*cked up all right — but not for a few days, a few weeks, even a few months. Nope. For years she raked in the cash through her wellness 'business', she raked in the cash by defrauding people and charities that didn't know she was collecting on their behalf, and they didn't see a cent.

But the very worst thing that Belle did, by telling them how to 'save their own lives', was to rob people of the months and maybe years of life they might have had if they took the conventional path and time offered by cancer treatments that, while toxic, are proven to work.

And that is an absolute tragedy.

Belle Gibson was once asked what advice she would give to people thinking about starting their own business. 'To have a point of difference,' she replied, 'to solve a problem or serve a purpose. All of these things are the crux of great business, but specifically a great app.'

Gibson rewrote her own history. She was one of the first health-and-wellness poster girls born on Instagram, legitimised on social media, and wildly successful on a global scale. But she is better known now as a cancer scammer than she could ever have dreamed of becoming as an app developer. She will go down in the history books as one of the biggest internet fraudsters of our time.

Many of Gibson's former friends and acquaintances were entrepreneurs in health and wellness-related fields. Most refused to speak to us for this book. 'I do not want to be associated with Belle Gibson or The Whole Pantry in any way' was a common refrain. These are the people who posed for photos with Gibson on Instagram, endorsed her, aligned themselves with her, and are named in the back of her book as being mentors and closest allies. But most said nothing; they would neither defend nor criticise her. Some of the more well-known figures actively discouraged anything being written by us about their links to Gibson. They tried to muddy the facts, and asked for commitments they would not be named in these pages. Some threatened legal action. *We trusted her. She took advantage of us. She has caused irreparable damage to this industry*, they said. And that is true. But what's also true is that the individuals who built Belle Gibson up are also partly responsible. They aligned themselves with her for their own benefit. 'She'd always have a few hangers-on, a little entourage,' said a source. When everything unravelled, most of the people who were so eager to bask in Gibson's glow suddenly disappeared. They, too, scrubbed clean their social-media profiles, erasing evidence of their friendship. But they helped to create her. Before she was on the front cover of magazines and flown around the world, she was just a young person who told lies on the internet. What might have evolved into a business by accident could most certainly have been stopped earlier had someone close to her asked the right questions.

While there was no doubt a failure of due diligence on many levels, Belle Gibson's allure cannot be understated. For a while, she was untouchable, a one-woman force. A former friend tries to explain how much power she wielded during her 18-month reign. 'So much that people outside the community cannot even fathom,' they said. 'People are still scared of her, scared of what the association with her will do to them, even years on. The fact that we're still scared gives her power. I imagine that she'd be enjoying this right now.'

The front door opens. Behind the flywire, the old woman looks puzzled. Her skin is soft, and her long hair, wispy-white, is tied up in a scrunchie. She's wearing black pants, a floral blouse, and maroon slippers. She doesn't want to talk about Belle Gibson. 'No, thank you,' she says. But a bad joke told on her doorstep puts her at ease.

She laughs, leans against the wall, and then unlocks the security screen. 'I think she's very clever, don't you?' she asks, with a wry smile. 'You better come in then.'

The woman is in her 80s. She lives in the ground-floor unit of a large, well-kept complex in an affluent suburb in Melbourne's east. She moved here about 10 years ago, after her husband died of cardiomyopathy. She'd met him under the steps of Melbourne's iconic Hotel Australia on Collins Street, which, in its heyday in the 1940s and 1950s, was one of the city's smartest society hotels. At the time, she worked at the Collins Book Depot, a small newsagency founded in 1922 that grew into the national chain Collins Booksellers. He was a book buyer for a department store. She has always loved reading and following current affairs. For decades, she's had Melbourne's *Age* newspaper delivered to her door each morning. That's how she found out that her granddaughter faked cancer and made a fortune.

The kitchen is spotless, and the carpets have fresh vacuum tracks, but she still apologises for the mess. Mid-afternoon sun slants through the custom-made curtains, which hang perfectly behind a pelmet, and fall onto the softly furnished sitting room. She is well-mannered and well-spoken, a hallmark of old time hospitality. She offers to turn down the chilly air conditioning, and later apologises for not having offered tea.

All around her comfortable home are photos of family: her five children, 14 grandchildren, and four great grandchildren. They're of weddings and birthdays and babies in baths. 'A shrine to my grandchildren,' she says, shuffling down the hallway toward the bedroom. Inside is a white French-provincial dresser next to an armchair, where three antique dolls with crimped hair and tailored outfits have been carefully placed. A couple of teddies and plastic dolls rest on another chair across the room. Gibson's grandmother walks towards two large photo collages that hang over a single bed. She straightens their silver-and-gold-rimmed frames, and talks through some of the pictures. Her finger stops on a cut-out of a younger her, taken in the early 1990s, holding a baby aged no more than 18 months. 'That's little Belle,' she says. 'I only saw her when she was a little girl. When I was her grandmother.'

She says the photo was taken when Gibson lived with her in Melbourne. She made the one-hour flight to Tasmania, and brought her back. She can't remember exactly how long her granddaughter stayed for; it could have been three months, or maybe six. 'I brought her back for a holiday because I love grandchildren,' she says, softly. 'She only just started to toddle at my house.' Then, one day before Christmas, she says Gibson's mother, Natalie, turned up with her older brother, Nick, and took her back. Since then, her contact with Gibson has been scant: the odd phone call from her granddaughter when she moved to Perth; a letter with a $5 note folded inside so Gibson could buy a coffee with her new friends. Gibson is estranged from her own mother, Natalie, so the old woman keeps tabs on her granddaughter through the media, despite living only 10 kilometres away, on the other side of town.

'I don't know anything about it, other than I know it's deceitful and wrong,' she says of Gibson's cancer scam. 'All the things that I taught my grandchildren, and children … and then a story comes along and knocks you down, and you just want to cuddle her up in your arms and wonder why-y-y-y … why someone would choose to have cancer when so many people …. how an idea comes to you about that?'

In the sitting room, Gibson's grandmother lowers herself backwards into a mechanical armchair a few feet from the television. Next to her on a small table is the day's newspaper, turned inside out, and a glossy magazine. While she talks, she kneads the muscle above her right knee. 'Bad osteoporosis,' she says, rubbing up along the side of her leg. She apologises for fidgeting. 'This is the last hip that was done, and I've had a fall.'

She switches from admiration for her 'intelligent' granddaughter to empathy with her victims, from urging she be punished for her actions to casting sole blame and culpability at the companies that put Gibson on a pedestal. A grandmother's love and mercy and tenderness for one of her own comes through strongly, but so does a sense of duty to protect the rest of her clan. She doesn't want them dragged into this mess. There's a feeling that the head of this family and everyone else cut Gibson loose long ago.

Asked if any relatives have been in touch with Gibson to offer support or advice since the spotlight was focused on her, she shakes her head slowly. Does the family talk about her? 'No. It's a forbidden subject,' she says. 'Of course, this worries all the other grandchildren. Supposedly they don't know about such things, but word creeps around that she's done wrong by cancer patients, and that would be the worst thing you could do in the world.' She sighs. 'To have no qualms about what is wrong and right … it is a concern.'

The grandmother says her family is respectable; her father was a policeman in country Victoria, and her children and their children have good jobs and run successful businesses. But Gibson's mother has always been the black sheep — vivacious, outgoing, a storyteller, and a trouble-maker. The old woman calls her Louise, the name she gave her at birth, not Natalie, the name her daughter changed it to later. She says Louise was one of the twins; the one who always attracted drama.

She shakes her head slowly, and tells stories about her daughter's parenting style, about the Salvation Army social workers who visited her when she was a young single mum living in public housing in Queensland. She says her other adult children get frustrated when she talks to Natalie on the phone. They want her to block the number, but she won't because she loves all her kids. But it's tough love.

'Louise rang me a couple of weeks ago and went on and on and said, "Now I've got cancer, I've only got three months to live." And I said, "Don't be ridiculous, we don't have cancer in our family." And I said the same to her when she said Belle had cancer. I said it can't be, because we don't have cancer in the Smillie family. I said, "Louise", "Natalie" — whatever she likes to call herself — "you can't say that. Have you got a diagnosis, a written diagnosis, and what are they doing for it?" She said, "Well there, I'm the first again."'

It's during conversations like these that Gibson's grandmother ponders how her granddaughter got into the terrible mess she's in. She says out loud what many others have speculated: 'Either [it] was learned behaviour, from her mother, or it's mental. But how could that be proved without her being assessed,' she asks, hopelessly. 'We don't know why. You could write a book on why. Why Belle? Does she know why?'

What she wants is for Gibson to focus on being a good mother. She says she should acknowledge what she has done, try to make it right, and allow people to give her a second chance. 'Take your child to school, and do tuckshop duty and all the things we did, mind other people's sick kids,' she says, 'and keep a low profile.'

As always with Belle Gibson, there are rumours about what she will do next, about how she will reinvent herself. She is still active on Snapchat. The people who follow that account say that she's been posting comments about launching her own dating app.

ACKNOWLEDGEMENTS

We feel incredibly privileged to have had the support of our families, friends, and co-workers, who have encouraged and sustained us throughout the writing of this book. A very special thank you to Kim and Grace, our beautiful partners, for your patience and forgiveness, and to our wonderful parents: Mary, who spent long nights armed with a marker, masterfully working her magic, and Rob and Joe, who read over every word. Many thanks, too, to our trusted readers, for their edits and feedback: Nicole Haddow, Priya Donelly, Louis Bowden, Caz Pringle, Nadege Hamdad, Jane Hutchinson, Jake Rausz, Sharon Donelly, Emily Malcolm, Gai Moritz, Chris Vedelago, and Jill Stark. Your critiques of the manuscript have made our work infinitely better.

To Kate Thomas and Monique Watt, two sincere and courageous women, thank you for allowing us into your lives for the best part of a year and for trusting us with your stories. And to all the people afflicted by cancer — and their families — who bravely spoke to us for this book, we are forever indebted to you. Our gratitude

324 THE WOMAN WHO FOOLED THE WORLD

also to the experts and interviewees who not only made themselves available, but generously took the time to answer our many, many follow-up questions.

To Eileen Berry, thank you for hounding us to look into the rumours that an Australian woman was faking cancer. Special thanks to Alex Lavelle, and to our editors, Michelle Griffin and Mat Dunckley, who have been wholly supportive of this project every step of the way, and to *The Age*, for allowing us the time to write away from the demands of the newsroom.

For their wisdom and advice and help, we would like to thank our colleagues Jason Steger, Konrad Marshall, Gina McColl, Kate Cole-Adams, Noel Towell, and Chloe Booker. And to our dear friends, Andrew Westman, John Wilson, Jaimee Mahony, Rebecca Thistleton, Stephen A. Russell, Rania Spooner, Julian Burak, Christine Irvine, and Paul Morris, we are so grateful for your endless encouragement.

Lastly, a very big thank you to the team at Scribe, in Australia and the UK, for bringing this book to life. To our incredibly supportive publisher, Henry Rosenbloom, who wholeheartedly believed this story should be told, thank you for your unwavering faith in us.